Praise for *Turn Autism Around*

*'If your child has no words, few words, or is showing any kind of delays, Mary's book will help, while also providing step-by-step instructions for potty training, feeding, tantrums, and more.'*

— **Temple Grandin PhD**, author of
*The Way I See It* and other books

*'It's been amazing to watch Mary's mission to turn autism around for millions. This book will be life-changing for many children and families around the world.'*

— **Jeff Walker,** author of the #1
*New York Times* bestseller *Launch*

*'As a professor of brain and cognitive science and the mother of twins born at 24 weeks, I deeply appreciate Dr. Barbera's commitment to serving and empowering scared parents who are looking, not just for answers, but for a roadmap. Dr. Barbera takes parents out of the position of waiting on experts in a broken medical system and gives them the tools they need to begin helping their children* now. Turn Autism Around *is absolutely essential reading.'*

— **Dr Susan Peirce Thompson**, *New York Times*
bestselling author of *Bright Line Eating*

*'Dr. Barbera's book lays out a nice sequence of 'what to do' for a child with autism or signs of autism, presented by someone who really knows what to do. The timing of this book is perfect.'*

— **Mark L. Sundberg PhD, BCBA-D**, author of the *VB-MAPP*

*'As a parent of a newly diagnosed toddler on the spectrum, I have to say that the advice and strategies in this book have been absolutely life-changing for our family. My 2-year-old daughter, Elena, is living proof that remarkable progress can be made in those precious months of 'waiting'. This is a must-read for any parent who is concerned about developmental delays in their child.'*

— **Michelle C.**, parent of Elena (a toddler featured in the book)

*'Mary Barbera has written the how-to, 'action guide' for parents concerned about their child's development. Filled with personal anecdotes from her journey, Barbera provides practical, research-based ideas for navigating those first few years of an autism diagnosis and her recommendations will no doubt help families feel less alone and empower them to help their child.'*

— **Dr Bridget Taylor PsyD, BCBA-D**,
co-founder and CEO of Alpine Learning Group

'When my daughter began displaying speech, behavior, and socialization difficulties before the age of 3, I didn't know what to do. I knew something was going wrong with my child, and fortunately, I stumbled across a treatment that helped her. As it turns out, not waiting for a diagnosis was the best thing I could've done. That was lucky. But it shouldn't be about luck. And now, it doesn't have to be! This is the guidebook that I wish I'd had, and that so many parents desperately need.'

— **Julie Ann Cairns**, mom and author of *The Abundance Code*

'This book is full of useful resources and helpful strategies to improve learning and decrease interfering behaviors. The forms, guidelines, and practical examples should be immensely helpful for those working with individuals who need support with areas such as communication, socialization, behavior, and daily living.'

— **Lynn Kern Koegel PhD**, Clinical Professor, Stanford University School of Medicine

'Mary's information in her new book Turn Autism Around *is life-changing for any parent noticing delays in their children. Following her easy, step-by-step action plans set me on a path to help my boys. If you want to turn hopeless into hopeful and empowered, this book is for you!'*

— **Kelsey G.**, autism mom to two boys featured in the book

'I have been fortunate to have known Dr. Mary Barbera for close to 20 years and have seen firsthand the positive impact of her work. In Turn Autism Around, *she shares the wealth of her experience to families who may be feeling incredibly scared and alone. Not only does she help parents and family members understand the power of early intervention, but she also empowers them to effectively deliver it.* Turn Autism Around *is that rare book which provides a ton of information and recommendations without being overwhelming or intimidating.'*

— **Michael J. Murray MD**, director, Division of Autism Services and Department of Psychiatry, Penn State Health

'Turn Autism Around *is a detailed book that provides parents with actionable steps that will allow their children to learn and thrive. Mary empowers parents to be 'the captain of the ship' on their child's journey to increased communication, skills, and happiness!'*

— **Rose Griffin SLP, BCBA**, owner of ABA Speech

'Mary Barbera's book and program empowered my family to begin turning autism around. While waiting for a diagnosis and eventual professional help, I was given the tools to begin teaching my grandson to communicate and shape his behaviors. Mary's approach is easy to learn and helped this grandma move mountains in the progress and development of our grandson.'

— **Diane H.**, 'gung-ho' grandmother

'Mary Barbera's action guide, Turn Autism Around, is the perfect 'first responder' resource for parents who are seeing the early signs of autism and who must make critical decisions concerning intervention and educational programming. It gives parents practical tools and strategies that they can begin to use immediately, even prior to the completion of formal assessments, thus taking advantage of precious intervention time that otherwise might be squandered.'

— **Gary S. Mayerson**, attorney and author of Autism's Declaration of Independence

'While showcasing the power behind the science of behavior analysis, Dr. Mary Barbera teaches parents how to implement fun, child-friendly interventions, even without access to well-trained professionals. These techniques, as outlined in her book, will have positive, life-long effects for your child, enabling you to take your power back as a parent.'

— **Amanda N. Kelly PhD, BCBA-D, LBA**, aka Behaviorbabe

'This book effortlessly covers the wide array of child development domains that exist for all children from play to sleep and everything in between. We live in a time where many of us parents feel lost and frustrated and this book gives us all an opportunity to re-connect with confidence and lessen the stress of the day-to-day toll of society.'

— **Megan Miller PhD, BCBA-D, LBA**, author and founder of Do Better Collective

'Turn Autism Around is practical, empowering, optimistic, and highly readable. It takes its place among the small but growing number of valuable contemporary science-based resources for parents of children with autism.'

— **William L. Heward EdD, BCBA-D**, professor emeritus, College of Education and Human Ecology, The Ohio State University

# TURN
# **AUTISM**
# AROUND

## ALSO BY DR MARY LYNCH BARBERA

*The Verbal Behavior Approach: How to Teach
Children with Autism and Related Disorders*

# TURN
# AUTISM
# AROUND

## An Action Guide *for* Parents *of* Young Children *with* Early Signs *of* Autism

**MARY LYNCH BARBERA** PhD, RN, BCBA-D

**HAY HOUSE**

Carlsbad, California • New York City
London • Sydney • New Delhi

**Published in the United Kingdom by:**
Hay House UK Ltd, The Sixth Floor, Watson House,
54 Baker Street, London W1U 7BU
Tel: +44 (0)20 3927 7290; Fax: +44 (0)20 3927 7291; www.hayhouse.co.uk

**Published in the United States of America by:**
Hay House Inc., PO Box 5100, Carlsbad, CA 92018-5100
Tel: (1) 760 431 7695 or (800) 654 5126
Fax: (1) 760 431 6948 or (800) 650 5115; www.hayhouse.com

**Published in Australia by:**
Hay House Australia Ltd, 18/36 Ralph St, Alexandria NSW 2015
Tel: (61) 2 9669 4299; Fax: (61) 2 9669 4144; www.hayhouse.com.au

**Published in India by:**
Hay House Publishers India, Muskaan Complex, Plot No.3, B-2,
Vasant Kunj, New Delhi 110 070
Tel: (91) 11 4176 1620; Fax: (91) 11 4176 1630; www.hayhouse.co.in

Text © Mary Lynch Barbera PhD, RN, BCBA-D, 2021

*Project editor:* Melody Guy • *Indexer:* J S Editorial, LLC
*Cover design:* Howie Severson • *Interior design:* Joe Bernier

The moral rights of the author have been asserted.

A catalogue record for this book is available from the British Library.

Tradepaper ISBN: 978-1-78817-696-5
Hardback ISBN: 978-1-4019-6147-3
E-book ISBN: 978-1-4019-6148-0
Audiobook ISBN: 978-1-4019-6149-7

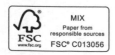

Printed and bound in Great Britain by
TJ Books Limited, Padstow, Cornwall

*I dedicate this book to my sons,*
*Lucas and Spencer, who taught me:*

*There is no such thing as "normal."*

*Life is not a sprint . . . it's a*
*marathon on a roller coaster.*

*And finally . . . there is no finish line*
*for me as a parent. I will never*
*stop learning how to be a better*
*teacher, advocate, and mom.*

*I love you both!*

# CONTENTS

When I was three years old, my mother realized there was something wrong with me. I did not talk or behave like the little girl who lived next door. When the grown-ups around me talked fast, it sounded like gibberish. I thought adults had their own special language. I remember feeling frustrated that I couldn't communicate, so I screamed and had tantrums.

Autism wasn't widely recognized in 1949 when I was two, so I was first labeled "brain damaged" by a neurologist who suggested my mother get a speech therapist to teach me to talk. Mother also hired a nanny to help keep me engaged all day long. She even figured out how to prevent my tantrums and learned how to teach me to wait and take turns with games. And because she didn't give up on me, I became fully verbal.

I always loved art and animals, and these interests were encouraged from an early age thanks to my mother and teachers. I went on to earn a degree in psychology and a Ph.D. in Animal Science. I have been a professor of Animal Science at Colorado State University for many years and, through my inventions and work, have made significant improvements in the cattle industry.

Because of my autism books, the conferences where I have spoken, and an Emmy Award–winning movie about my life, some people have called me the most famous autistic person in the world. Many times, parents ask me what to do when they have a two- or three-year-old child who is not talking or who is showing other signs of autism, and it may be a year before they can get either a diagnosis or professional services. I try to give them hope, holding myself up as an example of what's possible.

But most importantly, I tell them they have to act quickly and teach their child early. I'm a big believer in lots of early intervention for little kids with delays. The therapy is usually very similar for autism, speech delay, or sensory processing disorder. The worst thing you can do is to wait and do nothing.

Mary Barbera's book will show you how to start these interventions with or without an autism diagnosis. It will be really helpful to any parent with a young child who is not talking or having other developmental delays. Mary is a mom to a son with severe autism, a nurse, and a behavior analyst, so she understands how to help moms of young kids. Throughout the book, you will read about her transition from an overwhelmed parent to an autism professional.

One of the strategies Mary recommends in the book is saying words slowly and in a fun and animated way. She also encourages parents and therapists to pair words with objects and pictures. The combination of slowing words down and pairing words with visuals really worked for me, and it has worked for many other children.

If your child has no words or few words or is showing any kind of delays, this book will help. Parents also ask me all the time how to deal with potty training, feeding, sleep, tantrums, and more. Mary's book will give you step-by-step instructions for all of these issues.

You already suspect your child has a problem, so somebody needs to start working with him or her now. Mary's book shows that this "somebody" can be you.

—Temple Grandin, Ph.D., author of
*The Way I See It* and other books

# CHAPTER 1

# Early Signs of Autism Are an Emergency—So Why Are We Waiting?

If you've picked up this book, it's likely that you are stressed, overwhelmed, and worried about concerning delays in your child. Even worse, you might be frustrated with a long wait for an evaluation or intervention services. And if your child is already diagnosed with autism, you might be feeling angry that there is no one offering you ways to make things better. Whether you feel helpless against out-of-control tantrums, worried about your child's lack of speech, or confused because your pediatrician or therapists aren't giving you answers—I understand. As a parent, I've been there, too.

Perhaps you've even asked yourself:

*Is my child just strong willed?*

*Is my child simply a late talker who will catch up on their own?*

*Is this an early sign of ADHD?*

*Is this the dreaded A-word—autism?*

*Is there something I can do to help my child, regardless of the diagnosis?*

After more than 20 years as an international autism expert and a mother to a son with this diagnosis, I have had enough. The system for detecting and treating the earliest signs of autism and other developmental disorders is broken. And it breaks my heart to see so many families struggling and not knowing what to do.

The lines are far too long to see the right professionals for evaluations. And even if your child is already diagnosed with autism, you're likely still in line waiting to get to the right therapy or treatment. But there's some good news: you don't have to wait. In fact, *you should not.*

These may be the most important sentences you'll read in this book:

*Speech and social delays (which are often the earliest signs of autism) are an emergency.*

*You do not need a diagnosis or a team of professionals to begin treatment.*

*It's important to teach our children to communicate and reduce problem behaviors before they fall further behind.*

Here's what most parents don't know: Developmental disorders are quite common. In fact, 1 in 6 children ages 3 to 17 (or 17.8 percent) have a diagnosis of one or more developmental disorders,[1] including attention deficit hyperactivity disorder (ADHD), autism spectrum disorder (ASD), cerebral palsy (CP), hearing loss, intellectual disability (ID), learning disorders, and speech and language disorders. So if you're worried about a speech delay, attention issues, or excessive tantrums in your young child, you do have reason to worry, and you are not alone.

In addition to the alarming rate of developmental disorders, the autism rate has skyrocketed and now affects approximately 1 in 50 children. When my son Lucas was diagnosed in 1999, the autism rate was 1 in 500. In the 1970s, autism was thought to occur in 1 in 10,000, as illustrated by the following graph. There is much debate as to why so many of our children are being diagnosed with autism, ADHD, and other developmental disorders, but it's clear that the numbers are staggering.

In my work over the last two decades as a Board Certified Behavior Analyst at the doctoral level (BCBA-D), I've seen a global

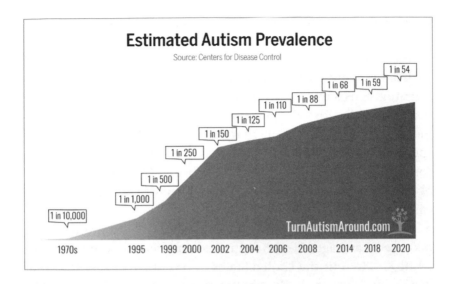

health emergency arise. While the rates of autism and other developmental disorders have drastically increased, there's a critical shortage of health care providers—namely, developmental pediatricians, neurologists, child psychiatrists, and specially trained psychologists—who can evaluate and diagnose children with autism. It can take nine months to two years to get an appointment for an evaluation to determine if it's "just" a delay or if it's something more serious such as autism or ADHD. And since the symptoms of all developmental disorders often overlap, some doctors who evaluate children when they are very young tell parents to wait another six months before returning. I also know of many kids who get the wrong diagnosis (the doctor says it's "just a delay" when it's actually autism) or multiple diagnoses over time. For example, a child might get a diagnosis of speech delay and sensory processing disorder (SPD) at two years, ADHD at four years, and autism at six years of age.

In the vast majority of cases, parents are forced to wait and worry. Can you imagine a scenario in which you were worried your child might have cancer, and the pediatrician was concerned enough to refer you to an oncologist . . . but you had to wait nine months for an evaluation? Then once you were given the cancer diagnosis, you had to wait longer for chemotherapy to start? It is heart wrenching to see families waiting as children are denied early and accurate diagnoses and treatment.

According to research, on average, children aren't diagnosed with autism until they are four or five years old, even though warning signs show up years earlier. The reality is that about 50 percent of all kids with autism don't get any therapy or treatment until they start elementary school. By that time, many of them have severe language and behavioral disorders and, in some cases, intellectual disability (with IQs below 70). This is primarily because their autism symptoms haven't been detected and treated early enough.[2]

Sadly, the situation is much more critical for children of color because on average, they're diagnosed and treated even later than white children in the United States. A recent paper reported that 27 percent of white children with autism spectrum disorder (ASD) also had intellectual disabilities (ID), while 47 percent of African American children and 36 percent of Hispanic children with ASD also have ID.[3]

At recent lectures I attended, as well as in a paper published in 2020 that he wrote with colleagues, Dr. Ami Klin has said that while autism traits are highly genetic, if children with delays or signs of autism are treated very early, intellectual disabilities, language disorders, and the problem behaviors that often accompany severe autism can sometimes be prevented or lessened in severity. Dr. Klin and the co-authors suggest that this is best done by not waiting for a diagnosis of autism before training parents on ways to repair the social interactions and back-and-forth communication between a parent and child as soon as they get off track.[4]

Additional research shows that if autism is caught early enough and treated intensively, some children can recover or become indistinguishable from their typically developing peers.[5] According to the Interactive Autism Network at Kennedy Krieger Institute, two large nationwide studies show that 4 to 13 percent of children lose their autism diagnosis by age 8 but often do keep other diagnoses such as language delay or ADHD.[6] *Children diagnosed before 30 months with less severe symptoms had the highest chance of recovery from autism.*

When my own son Lucas started showing signs of autism in the late 1990s, I knew almost nothing about autism, and I didn't realize that I was the one who needed to take action to help him. I also didn't know that turning autism around was even a possibility. Now I'm on a mission to change the outcome for all kids with autism or those just showing signs.

## A NOTE ABOUT GENDER USE AND CONFIDENTIALITY

Boys are four times more likely to be diagnosed with autism than girls.[7] For this reason, I will refer to children in this book as "he" and "his." Similarly, since the majority of primary caregivers, teachers, and therapists to young children with autism are female, I'll refer to the reader as "she" and "her." This is just to simplify the writing process and in no way negates the needs of young girls diagnosed with or showing signs of autism or the amazing caregiving and advocacy of men in the autism world.

I will also refer to you as the reader with the assumption that you're the mother of a toddler or preschool child between the ages of one and five who has either been diagnosed with autism or is showing signs of the disorder. But this book will also help if you're an early intervention or other type of professional who works with children of any age who are not conversational (and have the language ability of a young child under age five), as well as children who struggle with problem behaviors or difficulties with sleeping, eating, and potty training. The strategies work well for typically developing infants, toddlers, and preschoolers, too. So if you know, work with, or love a child age one through five (chronologically and/or developmentally) with or without delays, what you'll learn here will help you turn things around.

Note, too, that some of the families and children discussed throughout the book have requested that their names be changed to respect their privacy.

# THREE DANGEROUS MYTHS

There are three key dangerous myths in the world of autism and developmental delays that keep parents from getting their child the intervention they need.

## Myth 1: Your child's future is out of your control, and there's no hope for a "normal" life. So you have no choice but to wait.

The truth is that if you intervene now, your child *can* make significant improvements and possibly even avoid a diagnosis of autism and/or intellectual disability. But one thing I've learned over the years is that there is no such thing as a "normal" child; each human being has their unique strengths and challenges.

## Myth 2: You need a team of professionals, an official diagnosis, and/or insurance coverage to begin treatment.

You don't have to wait for any of those things. You can and should start today in your own home, using materials that you already have. You don't need a diagnosis or professionals to get started helping your child. You only need to assess his needs, and I'll provide simple tools for you to do that. If your child already has a diagnosis and a team of professionals on board, you still need this information. My Turn Autism Around (TAA) approach can be used by anyone, anywhere—with no experience or educational degree necessary. The strategies work because my step-by-step system is based on the science of applied behavior analysis (ABA) and B. F. Skinner's analysis of verbal behavior both of which have decades of research backing them up. Even better, my methods are child-friendly, fun, and easy to implement.

## Myth 3: There isn't enough time in the day to make a difference.

With just 15 minutes of simple exercises each day, you can change the trajectory of your child's life. You don't have to start with 20 to 40 hours of therapy per week (at least not right away) to teach your child and begin to catch up on their developmental delays.

# THE TURN AUTISM AROUND APPROACH

Research shows that some kids can lose their autism diagnosis and even the most severe forms of autism (with accompanying cognitive and behavioral disorders) can sometimes be made milder. I have personally seen this many times. I know of families who truly believe that by using the Turn Autism Around approach, they have reversed speech delays, reduced major problem behaviors, and in many cases lessened the severity of their child's autism.

In my years as a BCBA-D, I have seen my unique approach work over and over again. I've treated children with or without a diagnosis who were so out of control with tantrums that they were unable to go out with their families to social events. Some were even kicked out of daycare or preschool. Yet, with my strategies, these children started to talk, point, respond to their names, and socialize within weeks . . . or *days* in some cases. Even kids who made little to no progress in traditional therapy for months or years made gains.

As a parent only and not in my professional role as a behavior analyst, I've also met families of older children who are typically developing even though many professionals thought these children had autism when they were very young. Of course, no one, including me, has a crystal ball. But it doesn't matter what you or professionals call it—everyone can change and learn. There is no finish line, and diagnosing and treating autism is complicated.

Some people say they don't believe in autism recovery and consider autism to be a gift. These advocates (who are usually fully conversational adults with high-functioning autism) suggest that we shouldn't try to change children or make them "fit into" our world. But my approach doesn't try to change a child's personality or take away what makes each child special. Instead, it empowers parents to help their children communicate, sleep better, eat healthier food, potty train more easily, and become calmer and happier. In the end, I want every child with or without a diagnosis of autism to reach their fullest potential and be as safe, happy, and independent as possible.

The information I will provide here is based on decades of research of applied behavior analysis (ABA) treatment for children with autism, as well as my experience over the past two decades of working with thousands of children with autism and related disorders. There are some key distinctions between my approach and more traditional ABA programs, however.

The Turn Autism Around approach is completely child-friendly and positive, focusing on the whole child, as well as the family, to boost everyone's quality of life. I don't recommend punishment or using force to make a child do anything, and I discourage the practice of letting a child "cry it out." Instead, I've used everything I've learned about ABA and behavioral psychologist B. F. Skinner's analysis of verbal behavior, as well as my experience as a nurse, a behavior analyst, and a parent. The result is a set of simple practices that I designed to put parents at the helm of their child's journey as the "captain of the ship."

Let me tell you about some of the children who have made major progress. My client Faith went from lying on the floor screaming as many as 10 times per day as a two-year-old to thriving in a three-year-old daycare classroom at age three without any problem behaviors. Another client named Andrew transformed from having no words at all to talking in short phrases one year later.

Even children I've never met have made significant gains. Parker's parents were concerned that he wasn't speaking, but after learning my approach online and implementing the strategies, they watched him start to talk spontaneously in a matter of weeks.

A little boy named Chino was one of my most memorable clients. When I first met him, he was 20 months old, and out of hundreds of clients I'd worked with directly, he reminded me most of my son Lucas. When Lucas was 21 months old, my husband first suggested that he might have autism. But at that time, I didn't know about the effectiveness of early and intensive behavioral intervention, so Lucas didn't receive the right help as early as he should have. Chino, on the other hand, started receiving my help before he was two and had a remarkable transformation.

When I met Chino's mother, she had three children under the age of three. She was overwhelmed and incredibly worried about Chino's delays, and she didn't know what to do. When she arranged for early intervention therapy, I was the therapist sent to her home.

When I met Chino, in addition to completing the assessments you'll learn about in Chapter 4, I also completed a standardized test, the Screening Tool for Autism in Toddlers (STAT). This interactive tool, developed by Dr. Wendy Stone, includes a set of 12 activities that measure a child's social communication skills and risk for autism. This assessment gives information about the child's strengths and needs, and it can be used to identify goals and activities to improve skills.

One of the STAT items assesses a toddler's interest and ability to play with a doll. When handed a doll along with a doll bed, chair, bottle, and cup, a typically developing two-year-old will pick up the doll, talk to her, pretend to feed her, give her a nap, snuggle with her, and do all of the things that adults do with their babies. But when I gave the doll to Chino during the assessment, he immediately dropped the doll by his side. He never looked at it, and for the entire 30-minute test, he didn't speak, didn't play, and didn't interact with me—or with any of the materials I used during the assessment. Chino was in his own little world. It was clear that he was showing signs of autism and needed immediate help.

Six months later, Chino received a diagnosis of moderate-to-severe autism. Soon, his family received insurance funds for 20 hours a week of ABA therapy. I continued to work with them, teaching my methods of assessment, behavior intervention, and social skill development, while providing oversight of his ABA program. One year later—almost exactly to the day—after many hours spent using the tools and strategies included in this book, I repeated the STAT doll test with Chino. He had not seen the doll or any of my other assessment tools since that original test. This time, when I handed him the baby doll, he immediately put her in the bed and told her "night-night." He kissed her, woke her up, and then said, "All done night-night"—all while his mother wept tears of joy and relief. By second grade, Chino was fully conversational, bilingual, and in a mostly mainstream educational program at school. (For free book resources and to see videos of Chino's transformation, visit TurnAutismAround.com.)

## MY FALL INTO THE AUTISM WORLD

Although my son Lucas's symptoms looked just like Chino's at 20 months, his trajectory was quite different. Back then, when Lucas was a baby in the late 1990s, he was warm and cuddly with me but had little language and a quirky obsession with letters. I was pregnant with our second child, Spencer, when Lucas began to slowly regress and show signs of autism shortly after his first birthday. Very gradually, he stopped waving, stopped saying "hi" to people, stopped doing hand motions to songs, became a pickier eater, became more addicted to his pacifier and the TV, and had difficulty sleeping. As a first-time mom, I thought Lucas was just going through a phase. I was unaware that he was getting off track or regressing.

As he approached the 18-month mark, Lucas also had no awareness of the upcoming arrival of his baby brother. And after Spencer was born, my husband, Charles, an emergency medicine physician, became secretly alarmed by our son's failure to notice the new baby in our house. While I still didn't realize that Lucas's lack of awareness of his baby brother was an issue, looking back on that time, we could have replaced Spencer with a plastic baby doll, and Lucas would not have noticed.

A few months later, when Lucas was 21 months old, Charles dropped the bomb, saying the A-word for the first time. "Do you think Lucas has autism?" he asked me.

I was shocked and horrified, as I'd never thought there was anything wrong with Lucas. I looked at Charles and said, "I never *ever* want to hear the word *autism* again."

I didn't know much about autism, especially what it would look like in a toddler. I didn't know real treatment was available or that there was anything I could do to turn autism around, so I felt defensive immediately. *There's no point pinning this death sentence of a diagnosis on my toddler*, I thought.

For more than a year, Charles abided by my wishes and didn't bring it up. But the A-word had been etched into my brain. I thought about the possibility of autism when Lucas lost words or skills. I thought about autism when Lucas failed to start talking in phrases by age two despite starting toddler preschool and then speech therapy a few months later. I felt helpless as my son continued to fall further behind.

After more than a year of worrying on my own, praying it was anything but autism, I finally did some research and found out about hyperlexia, the ability to read letters and words before you can speak. Through that research, I met a woman who had a son with both autism and hyperlexia. She suggested I look into ABA therapy for Lucas, even though I thought he was just speech delayed. "If they're recovering kids with severe autism," she said, "treating your son with a speech delay should be easy."

The woman also recommended Catherine Maurice's 1993 book, *Let Me Hear Your Voice*. As soon as I started reading it, I recognized my son in the descriptions of autism. *Oh, my God*, I thought, *I've been in denial for over a year, doing nothing*. I had no idea there was any hope for children with autism, but this book, which outlined the power of ABA therapy, taught me that up to half of kids could "become indistinguishable" from typically developing kids with intensive behavioral intervention. As a result, I did an immediate about-face.

I got Lucas on a three-month waiting list for an evaluation at the Children's Hospital of Philadelphia. He was diagnosed the day before his third birthday.

Even though we were somewhat prepared, it was still devastating to get the definitive answer. Plus, Charles and I expected a diagnosis of mild autism, but when the developmental pediatrician came back with a moderate-to-severe diagnosis, it was my worst fear realized.

I asked about recovery using ABA, but the doctor wasn't optimistic. He explained that in his long career, he hadn't seen kids with Lucas's developmental delays catch up completely. While he didn't say it outright, my denial and delay in getting Lucas evaluated and treated had been a big mistake.

On the way home from the appointment, Lucas was completely silent. He was buckled into his car seat, staring out the window. No words, no babble. Just silence.

I cried as my husband ticked off the list of things Lucas would never do—*never go to college, never get married, never . . .*

"Please be quiet," I pleaded with him.

Even in my sadness, however, I clung to hope for recovery. It was what I was looking for, so I wasn't willing to give up that hope. I was going to work as hard as possible to help Lucas catch up as much as he could. I felt a lot of guilt about my denial. I talk about my "fall" into the autism world because it felt like I had fallen into a deep dark hole with Lucas. I had to figure out how to claw my way out of that hole and help my son because I knew his life depended on it.

I had no idea how to start, but I dug in completely. I got him therapists, and when I found out there weren't enough of them, that's when I became a behavior analyst myself so that I could help Lucas more, and eventually others.

From 2003 onward, I have worked with hundreds of kids directly, trained thousands of parents and professionals around the world, and educated pediatricians and health care practitioners on the early warning signs of autism. I started several groups to raise awareness about autism in general, and then more specifically to advocate for early diagnosis and early treatment. I wrote the book *The Verbal Behavior Approach: How to Teach Children with Autism and Related Disorders* about what I had learned. It has been used by parents, grandparents, therapists, and educators for more than a decade and is now available in more than a dozen languages.

In that book, however, I didn't talk much about catching the earliest warning signs of autism, prevention of the disorder, reversal of symptoms, or recovery. As I began to treat more and more children at younger ages, I saw hundreds of kids improve by leaps and bounds due to very early treatment. And some of them were just like Lucas when he first showed signs of autism at 21 months. This was especially true for children ages 1 to 5 who had at least one all-in, proactive parent by their side spring into action at the very first signs of delays and red flags.

My work made it clear that early intensive behavioral intervention using my Turn Autism Around approach also helped children diagnosed with only speech delays to catch up faster. The sooner children received treatment, the sooner some of them were able to reach the same developmental milestones as their peers. And those with autism who were unable to catch up completely with their typical peers were still able to make great strides. *Waiting simply puts children further and further behind.*

What about Lucas? Well, he made significant progress once he started an intensive ABA program and was transitioned into using the verbal behavior approach. But his treatment was delayed by my denial and subsequent waiting lists for almost two years from the time he started showing signs of autism. So his progress was steady . . . but slow.

I can't know for sure, of course, that earlier treatment would have made Lucas indistinguishable from his typical peers or that he would have progressed to the same degree as Chino. But I'm certain he would have made more progress if I hadn't wasted more than a year denying the possibility of autism.

I believe Lucas's life would be easier today with earlier intervention. As someone with moderate-to-severe autism and a mild intellectual disability, Lucas needs a lot of supervision and care. But he can request what he needs, take a shower, make his breakfast, tie his shoes, answer questions, sing songs, and more—all as a result of the right kind of treatment. My goal for Lucas now that he has reached adulthood is that he remains stable and as safe, independent, and happy as possible. This is the same goal I have for my younger son, Spencer, who is also an adult, and for all kids with or without autism.

This is why I have become such an advocate for empowering parents to take action and *not wait*. I want parents to have hope and not put their heads in the sand. Hoping that Lucas's issues would resolve themselves didn't turn autism around for him, and it won't for your child either.

Nevertheless, remember that "turning autism around" looks different for every child. The results will be some shade of gray rather than black or white. So I can't promise that a diagnosis of autism can be prevented or that your child's speech delay will be reversed. Your child may be like Lucas—already diagnosed with severe autism and an intellectual disability, which might mean lifetime care. Or your child may catch up completely and not receive any diagnosis. The ultimate diagnosis could be a speech delay, a learning disability, ADHD, or autism, and the diagnosis may change over time. Your child may simply be overly sensitive and have excessive tantrums. But regardless of the diagnosis or lack thereof, getting into high gear now will only make life better for you both. Using my child-friendly Turn Autism Around approach is helpful at any stage and any age, and getting ahead of the difficult behaviors and catching up with language and social skills are far more significant than the diagnosis.

## THE A-WORD

One thing you're going to have to get over is using the A-word. The woman who suggested Lucas try ABA even if he only had a speech delay gave me the permission I needed to look into autism.

The strategies outlined in this book should work when used by caregivers or professionals trying to help any young child with any social communication delays, sensory processing issues, severe tantrums or those having difficulties with sleeping, eating, potty training, or going into the community.

So if you've picked up this book and don't want to use or read the word *autism*, I get it.

But keep reading. Please.

# SIBLINGS, TWINS, AND MEDICAL ISSUES

You may be reading this book because you already have one child with autism, and you're concerned about delays or possible signs of autism in their younger siblings. Studies show that siblings have a 16 to 36 percent chance of having autism.[8] This means that at least one in five children who have an older sibling with autism will also be diagnosed. Siblings are also more at risk of having developmental delays that don't meet the autism diagnosis threshold. Nevertheless, the delays may present very differently in siblings, so parents who have one child with ASD often need to watch their younger children carefully for anything that may signal the need for early intervention—even if those behaviors are very unlike those of your older children. Sometimes, a younger child is diagnosed first, and then the family realizes that an older sibling has a milder form of the disorder.

There are sibling research studies at major institutions and hospitals. If you live close enough to one of them and you want professionals to help you closely monitor your baby for signs of autism, you can enroll newborn or infant siblings free of charge.

One of the direct benefits of enrolling a younger sibling in a study is that the researchers can complete developmental testing every few months and identify delays. This will allow you to start interventions as soon as possible if your baby shows delays.

I've worked with many families in which more than one child received a diagnosis of autism. I worked with one family that had three children with the diagnosis, although the signs and symptoms appeared very differently. The middle child, Jeremy, had the most significant needs. When I started working with him at age four, his IQ was below 70, and he was officially diagnosed with intellectual disability in addition to autism. After using my approach for a year, Jeremy's IQ went up by 30 points, and he was no longer intellectually disabled. In that same year, Jeremy became fully conversational and is now in traditional high school, has friends, is a star athlete, and is on track for college. His two siblings also did very well, and autism is no longer the primary diagnosis for any of them.

What about twins? Are they also both more likely to be diagnosed with autism? Research done on twins shows that there is a very strong genetic component involved, but even in identical twins, the rate of autism for both is not 100 percent, suggesting that there are environmental factors involved, too.

Here's another important point: my son and almost all my former clients with autism have had medical issues that may have contributed to or complicated their autism, including gastrointestinal issues (constipation, diarrhea, acid reflux), allergies, asthma, eczema, seizures, and autoimmune disorders, to name just a few. Even though I'm a registered nurse and married to a physician, the medical assessment and treatment of kids aren't my areas of expertise, so I won't cover them much in the book. But I will say this: your child needs a health care practitioner who doesn't discount medical issues or blame problems like diarrhea on autism or ADHD. If your child's pediatrician isn't open to addressing your child's medical needs, you may have to find specialists and/or a functional medicine practitioner who can guide you through the medical issues that could be contributing to your child's delays.

## TIME IS OF THE ESSENCE

The bottom line is that there is an epidemic of children waiting for both diagnosis and treatment. The average age for children to be diagnosed and begin treatment is now four or five years old. That's at least three years after you can use my approach to most effectively treat concerning behaviors and teach language and play skills.

*It really is an emergency for young children just showing signs.*

But if your child is older and/or has significant impairment, it's not your fault and it's okay not to panic or feel guilty. In my first book, I wrote that if it was all about how hard I worked, Lucas would no longer have autism. I now know that sometimes neurological damage is severe and permanent and this doesn't mean you failed your child or that he cannot make meaningful progress.

On the pages that follow, I will guide you through the Turn Autism Around approach. You'll receive help with eating, sleeping, potty training, speaking, imitating, play, safety, and eliminating problem behaviors. You'll meet people who have seen their children improve and a few for whom we feel confident a diagnosis of autism was prevented. You'll find out how to quickly assess your child's skills, create a plan, start teaching in small 15-minute sessions daily, find the right professionals, and advocate for your child.

So no matter the age of your child or his level of functioning right now, this book is for you. I want to empower you to move forward in becoming your child's best teacher and advocate for life. I want to equalize the playing field as much as possible by giving you and all parents around the world a clear path to begin detecting and treating autism and other developmental disorders as soon as you can.

You may be at the start of your journey up the mountain, or you may already be halfway up. You might have a short climb or be facing a long climb up a steep mountain. But no matter where you are on the mountain, I'm here to lead the way.

I know you can do it because more than 20 years ago, I was climbing that same mountain as a mom with a son who was given a diagnosis that terrified me. I had no map, so I had to make one. This book is that map.

If your child has problem behaviors, a speech delay, sleep problems, or anything that concerns you, start helping him now. Let's replace fear with hope and the status quo with progress. Let's help you become the most empowered and proactive parent you can be. Let's catch and treat the earliest signs of autism and change the trajectory of your child's life!

# CHAPTER 2

# Is It Autism, ADHD, or "Just" a Speech Delay?

When you feel your child may be falling behind his peers, it's natural to become confused. Is he delayed? Is this just the "terrible twos" that have started early or extended into the threes? Does he have autism? Will the issue "fix itself"?

Not only is there a range of "normal," but there are many factors that could cause a child to become delayed in one or more areas. Some kids are premature, so they are automatically delayed in some ways. Some have multiple siblings who model good or bad behaviors, and others are only children with no siblings. Plus, boys tend to talk a little bit later than girls.

Children with autism often have tantrums, but so do typically developing kids. And each child has his own personality and temperament. I remember saying that if my youngest son Spencer had autism, we would have had our hands full because he was always more sensitive and "higher maintenance" than Lucas, who had a laid-back personality from the beginning.

Many children with language or other delays do catch up, either on their own or with a little bit of early intervention therapy. Even children with high IQs and no developmental delays often have sensory and social differences from their peers. Meanwhile, some signs of autism and ADHD in toddlers are nearly identical, including inattention, hyperfocus on particular topics, hyperactivity, impulsivity, and refusing to wait, share, or take turns.

I've learned that there's a huge overlap between early signs of autism, ADHD, speech delays, and mental health disorders. To confuse matters even further, there's the issue of regression that I mentioned in Chapter 1 with the story of my son Lucas. Maybe your child used to wave, but suddenly he has stopped or almost never waves anymore. Maybe his language skills have regressed. Data from the Autism and Developmental Disabilities Monitoring Network estimates that at least 20 percent of children with autism experienced some loss of skills at some point in their development. One small study indicated that 86 percent of children who eventually receive a diagnosis of autism have a decline in social skills between the ages of six months and three years.[1]

So how on earth can you tell if what *your* child has is autism, ADHD, "just" a speech delay, or typical toddler tantrums? How can you be sure you need to take action?

This chapter will include a list of behaviors/symptoms to watch for. I know reading such a list can be disturbing, especially if you recognize your child in any of the descriptions. But it isn't definitive, and it isn't a diagnosis. The fact that you're reading this book means you're ready to be on top of action and advocacy for your child.

Whatever issues he faces, you're now on the verge of discovering what he needs. So remember: for every behavior/symptom on the list that follows, you will learn interventions and strategies throughout these pages to help him improve or possibly even alleviate that symptom.

Consider one of my former clients, Max. His family lived near the beach in New Jersey, and one day, at 15 months, he suddenly freaked out and wouldn't touch the sand. As he approached the 2-year mark, it was alarming for his parents that he couldn't talk, didn't make eye contact, and erupted in explosive tantrums many times a day. After a year of waiting and worrying, his mother got him an appointment for an assessment, but the doctors couldn't conduct the test because Max screamed uncontrollably for an hour and a half.

A month later, the family moved to Pennsylvania, and I became Max's early intervention therapist. During my initial meetings with him, he could say just one word—*pizza*—which he used for everything, even though his mother said he didn't like pizza. He demanded his bottle 10 times an hour and hit his mother whenever she said no. Soon after the move, Max failed the STAT screening test for autism. Because of this, his pediatrician believed that Max would be clinically diagnosed with it.

When he was two and a half years old, and had failed the STAT test, I started treating him over a four-month period for three hours a week, while also training his mother in the techniques I've created. The results were profound, and Max experienced a remarkable transformation. He began pointing and talking, and his tantrums decreased. As a result, he never received a diagnosis of autism. By age five, he was caught up developmentally and was typical in every way. He entered kindergarten without needing any services. His parents were relieved and overjoyed.

"Without Mary's help when Max was two," his mother says, "I'm almost positive he would have been diagnosed with autism, and we would have had a very different life."

Of course, as I made clear in Chapter 1, I can't promise everyone the same results as Max. But I do know that with the Turn Autism Around approach, many children can and do improve dramatically.

## WHAT IS AUTISM SPECTRUM DISORDER (ASD)?

Autism spectrum disorder refers to a developmental disorder with symptoms appearing usually by age three or before, although diagnoses can come much later. When children or adults are diagnosed, professionals often ask if there was a speech delay or repetitive interests in their early years.

Back when Lucas was diagnosed, the *Diagnostic and Statistical Manual of Mental Disorders* (DSM) was in version 4. At that time, pervasive developmental disorder (PDD-NOS), Asperger's syndrome (AS), and autistic disorder all fell under autism spectrum disorder. Now, with version DSM-5, everyone with these disorders is given the diagnosis of autism spectrum disorder (ASD). If you have a child who was previously diagnosed with Asperger's syndrome or PDD-NOS, no one's going to make you stop using those terms, but they are no longer individual diagnostic categories.

The DSM-5, which was published in 2013, categorizes autism into three levels. Those at Level 1 need just a little support, Level 2 needs more support, and Level 3 indicates severe autism with significant needs. These levels are pretty subjective, and an individual's level can definitely change over time. Your child could start out as a Level 3. Then with the right therapy, he could move to Level 1. I've seen this many times, especially if a child is labeled high or low at a young age. Children can also worsen over time, especially if delays are not caught early and treated. As you can see, autism is definitely a spectrum disorder.

There is a lot of talk in the autism world about low functioning versus high functioning. Many parents want to know if it's possible to predict how a two-year-old will do when he's older, and my answer to that question is no. Still, as I said in Chapter 1, it's true that a younger child with mild symptoms has a better chance of avoiding the diagnosis of autism or catching up with intervention. I've personally known many children who started out with very few skills and looked low functioning but went on to do very well. Some of my previous clients are learning to drive and going to college, for example.

While we can't predict how a child will do, we can give them the best possible chance of reaching their full potential by starting our interventions as early as possible.

## SIGNS TO WATCH FOR

The behaviors or symptoms that follow are red flags for autism, but again, please don't jump to conclusions and go into a panic. That said, if your child exhibits any of these, I urge you to take the actions I'll recommend later in the chapter.

Even if your child has already been diagnosed with autism, knowing these signs can help you assess him with regard to each symptom. That knowledge will help you set goals, understand what to teach him as you continue reading the book, and choose the best professionals to help him.

- **Pointing.** Even with my nursing background, when my son Lucas was young, I had no idea of the importance of pointing. Soon after he was diagnosed, I learned that a lack of pointing is a critical red flag for autism. When I assess an 18-month-old or a 2-year-old child, I first ask: Does the child point? It's also important for a child to respond to your pointing. For instance, if you point across the room to a stuffed animal or the TV and say, "Look, Johnny!" does the child's attention go in that general direction? When a child passes the 15- or 18-month mark, or certainly by age 2, he should be pointing with his index finger on a very regular basis. Children at this age should be pointing at things they want like juice or a toy, as well as pointing to show you things, such as an airplane flying above.

  Children can also stop pointing, which happened to Lucas around 15 months. After that, instead of pointing, Lucas would often take an adult's hand and place it on the item he wanted. This behavior is called "hand leading," and in addition to a lack of pointing and responding to pointing, it's another red flag for autism.

  Keep in mind, however, that some children with autism do point by 18 months, so while it's an important red flag, this alone isn't sufficient for a diagnosis. I once knew a speech and language pathologist (SLP) whose son was diagnosed with severe autism at age 3. The first sign for her came when he was a year old, and she noticed that he didn't have an interest in toys. Soon, she noticed language delays. When she mentioned her concerns during a pediatrician well visit, the doctor told her, "If he can point, he's not autistic." Quite simply, that doctor was wrong. But if your child isn't pointing by 18 months or 2 years old, it's important to take action and teach him this critical skill using the techniques you'll learn as you continue reading.

- **Speech and Language Delays.** Even before a child starts to speak, a baby or toddler should be smiling, babbling, and cooing at adults. This is the beginning of social language. Limited babbling, smiling, and attention toward faces could be an early red flag for autism in babies. Very young children should also begin to understand language.

   When Lucas was two, I had a photographer come to the house to take family pictures. The photographer gave Lucas a piece of trash and said, "Here, buddy, throw this away," but Lucas had no idea what the guy was talking about. The photographer was perplexed, obviously thinking my son was old enough to understand.

   At the time, I brushed it off because I didn't know if he should or shouldn't know such a thing at age two. I later found out that Lucas's inability to follow directions was related to his receptive language, which means his ability to understand language when others speak to him. A receptive language delay differs from an expressive language delay having to do with speech. It's important to determine if your child has an expressive language delay or talking problem and/or if he has difficulty understanding language. A mixed receptive and expressive language delay is much more common in young kids with autism.

Some children have speech, but it seems different or not functional. Maybe your child counts to 10 and can identify letters, but he won't get things when you ask him to retrieve them. Maybe he doesn't call you "Mom," or he frequently repeats lines from movies or things you've said. Landon was three when his mother, Nicole, started using my approach. He was talking in short phrases composed mostly of lines he memorized from movies, so a lot of his speech was repetitive. Both his language and play skills were off track for his age. Once Nicole started using my strategies, she was able to start turning around her son's defective and delayed language issues.

Then there are simpler problems that cause or contribute to speech delays like the overuse of pacifiers. Two-year-old Amy wasn't speaking much because she was addicted to her pacifier and constantly "plugged up." Her speech delay resolved when her mom learned my pacifier-weaning methods.

Some people blame speech delays on older siblings who talk for the younger child or on adults who are too quick to deliver what they think the child wants as soon as the tears start. Truthfully, these can be factors. As you continue reading, you'll learn more about how to assess whether or not your child has a speech and language delay and what you can do about it.

- **Excessive Tantrums.** Many typically developing children have tantrums, but children with autism have a tendency toward an excessive number of them. This is primarily due to their lack of communication skills. When a child can't communicate what he wants to the adults around him, he naturally becomes frustrated and may resort to tantrums. While *tantrum* is a relative term that may mean different things to different people, children with autism often whine, cry, scream, fall to the floor, or even become aggressive. Some kids might throw items, tear up paper, or write on walls, which is called "property destruction" in the ABA world. Some might even engage in self-injurious behavior (SIB) by hitting or biting themselves. If your child is engaging in any serious problem behaviors like severe aggression, property destruction, or SIB that's dangerous or life-threatening, you must seek medical care immediately. Even if your child isn't displaying any serious problem behaviors at this point, it's critical that you learn how to teach language and social skills to prevent these kinds of problems before your child grows bigger.

- **Not Responding to His Name.** This is another common red flag for autism. In fact, some kids who don't respond to their names are initially thought to be deaf, until they respond to some other sound. Ruling out hearing loss is important with any speech and language delay, but most young children with signs of autism tend to be in their own world and often have "selective hearing." I was concerned that Lucas had hearing loss when he was two, but a few days before the scheduled hearing test, he heard the theme song for a favorite TV show playing quietly and came running into the room to watch. As you continue reading the book, you'll learn methods for getting your child to respond to his name in an easy and fun way (even if he's already been diagnosed with autism).

- **Playing Behaviors.** I also look at playing behaviors as possible red flags. Does the child play with a variety of toys appropriately? Or is he very focused on one object or a set of objects that he needs to carry around all the time? Does he play with the same toys over and over, such as stacking blocks or lining up cars for several minutes or hours?

  Another subtest within the STAT screening tool involves handing a child a bubble container with the lid tightly closed. Most typically developing children will hand the bubbles back to you, while babbling and engaging in eye contact, trying to communicate to you that they need help in opening the jar. A child with autism may hand it back to you, but without eye contact or babbling, and might stare at your hand without looking at your face at all. Lack of eye contact during playful interactions can be one of the first signs of autism in babies and toddlers.

  By three or four years of age, most children will engage in sharing toys, playing games, and in pretend play throughout the day. While they play, they negotiate language back and forth with other children. Pretend play and an interest in peers are usually very delayed in children with autism. They might be stuck in parallel play mode, in which they play separately alongside other kids without playing with other kids, and they may struggle with sharing.

- **Repetitive Behaviors.** A child with autism may flap his hands in front of his face, line up objects, or engage in spinning his whole body or toys that aren't generally meant to be spun. I worked with one child who carried and hoarded figurines and another boy who rocked himself and banged his head on hard and soft surfaces throughout the day. But in some kids like Lucas, repetitive behavior wasn't so obvious. He liked to watch the same TV shows over and over but didn't have any other repetitive behaviors that were concerning early on.

In Chapter 1, I mentioned *hyperlexia*, the ability to recognize letters and read prior to the ability to speak. In some children, it manifests as an extreme interest in letters and numbers, obsessive rearranging letter blocks to spell words, or singing the alphabet song.

Some kids with more language may have a hyperfocus on trains, maps, watching the same YouTube clips repetitively, or as Landon did in the example earlier, repeating or "scripting" lines from movies.

- **Sameness.** An insistence on sameness might be an indicator, such as wanting to eat out of the same bowl, wear the same shirt every day, or always take the same route to the playground. Children with autism often don't like change, and they sometimes have tantrums when a change occurs because it causes them stress.

- **Sensory Issues.** Kids with sensory disorders and those with autism are often especially overreactive or underreactive to sensory stimuli. Some children have an aversion to bright lights, for example, and they overreact to the sense of sight. They may also be overreactive to sensory input, covering their ears or having tantrums when there are too many people around or when the environment is noisy. My son Lucas is bothered by noise and often wears headphones to drown out excessive sound.

  Yet, some kids can be underreactive to language and noise. For example, they might not respond to their name, as mentioned before.

  Some kids can't stand being touched. They may become overreactive because of the tags in clothing, which most of us don't even notice. Other kids are underreactive to touch and need heavy pressure. They often jump or seek input by running into walls or squishing themselves inside sofa cushions.

Children may have reactivity issues when eating, too. They might react to the sight, colors, tastes, textures, flavors, or temperatures of food. The way different brands of macaroni and cheese look can cause a reaction, for instance.

- **Motor Delays and Toe Walking.** Studies have shown that children with autism walk later on average than typically developing children, and some walk on their toes when they are young. Children with developmental delays and disorders also show fine motor delays and motor planning issues that can affect many self-help skills like buttoning clothing and using utensils. One of my clients, Cody (you'll hear more about him in Chapter 5), started before the age of one with physical therapy and occupational therapy for motor issues and was diagnosed with autism at 18 months of age.

- **Imitation.** Finally, imitation of simple actions usually begins around eight months, and by the age of two, most kids imitate everything. This is the way language and play typically develop. In almost all the young kids with autism I've treated, there has been a big delay with imitation.

If you recognize your child in any of the descriptions in this section, what should you do next? The most important thing is to avoid sticking your head in the sand like I did—even if your child seems to be mostly on track with only one or two delays. Like me, you might be getting false reassurance from family members and professionals, but the interventions in this book will help your child grow in his development. Even if you've been in denial for months or years like I was, don't beat yourself up. You're here now, and I'm going to be your guide to turning autism (or signs of autism) around starting today.

There are three key steps that I recommend parents take, whether your child already has a diagnosis, or you're just beginning to assess what's going on.

## THREE STEPS YOU CAN TAKE RIGHT NOW

Whether you're worried, on the waiting list for an evaluation, or your child has already been diagnosed and is even receiving multiple therapies at this point, you can take these steps to improve your situation.

### Step One: Finish reading this book and learn my approach.

This will give you a firm foundation to not only begin to work with and help your child at home, but to also better assess the professionals and therapies available to you. As you read the next chapters on safety and early assessments, strategies for specific behaviors, and advocacy, you will have a much better idea which professionals will help your child.

Early on in my career as a behavior analyst, I recommended that everyone see a pediatrician at the first signs of a developmental delay and that all children should be referred to early intervention and an ABA provider as soon as possible. I believed that ABA and any kind of early intervention services were better than none. Over the years, however, I've discovered this isn't true. I've learned all too well that any type of therapy, treatment, or professional can be good, mediocre, or even bad for your child.

The pediatrician who mistakenly brushed off the possibility of autism because a boy could point shows that many professionals just don't know enough. Well-meaning physicians, BCBAs, occupational therapists, speech language pathologists, family, friends, and more may give you (or have given you) contradictory—and often wrong—advice. I've heard about many professionals making statements to parents such as:

*Wait and see.*
*He needs the pacifier to soothe himself.*
*Just let him cry it out.*
*Put him in time-out if he hits you.*
*He needs daycare or preschool to socialize.*
*Don't worry; he'll catch up on his own.*
*Leave it all to the professionals.*

Unfortunately, all these statements can put you in the same place I was with my son: not taking important action at the first sign of delays. Or worse—receiving ineffective or even harmful therapies.

One of the moms in our online community drove more than an hour with her two-year-old to see a speech therapist. According to their "policy," she had to wait in the waiting room and wasn't allowed to accompany her son into the therapy room to watch and learn. She couldn't ensure that he was properly cared for or taught in a positive way. She was especially worried because he couldn't speak yet, and he screamed all the way into the room and throughout most of his sessions. When she brought up her concerns to the therapist, she was told to "go shopping" while her son received therapy. "He'll stop crying eventually," they told her. Soon after, she learned how to work with her son using the Turn Autism Around approach and stopped that long commute. He also stopped crying while he was being taught. *No child should cry or scream during therapy, and parents should be active participants in their child's learning. If the child hates the learning, something is wrong with the teaching method.*

In another instance, a parent spent a year consulting with very expensive therapists while her son cried throughout his sessions. His only progress in that 12-month period was learning how to clap. But he clapped when anyone said anything to him, not just the word *clap*. So this so-called progress wasn't actually progress.

Meanwhile, for an entire year, he associated learning with something he hated.

Unfortunately, very few parents and professionals know how to implement the Turn Autism Around approach. It can and should be layered on to whatever treatments you have available locally, especially if your child has a diagnosis of autism or goes on to get one. Once you learn my approach, you'll be the "captain of the ship," and you'll know what therapy and which professionals your child needs next month, next year, and beyond.

Throughout the chapters, you'll learn a great deal about what your child needs in terms of therapy and how to choose the best team for him. You'll also learn how to best advocate for him. Before that more in-depth discussion, however, I want to give you just a few advocacy tips to get you started:

- You've probably heard the phrase "Don't burn your bridges." Well, I recommend keeping this in mind as you enter the world of autism intervention and advocacy. Avoid an "us versus them" mentality. You need to be assertive and smart, but not aggressive.

- Your child's plan and goals should be based on his skills. I've seen therapists try to get children to perform tasks that were far beyond their current capacity. There's no time for goals about learning prepositions, pronouns, or colors if your child isn't articulating his basic needs.

- You need to learn how to teach your child. Only then will you truly have the power to stop relying exclusively on the opinions of others.

- The focus should be on *your* child. When there are too many opinions, and you become confused, step back and observe him. Then pick the option that's best for him.

## Step Two: Learn typical developmental milestones and compare them to your child's development.

The Centers for Disease Control and Prevention (CDC) website includes an index of developmental milestones in terms of language, self-care, self-regulation (ability to calm themselves down), and other areas. Of course, no two children are the same, so the index just offers an age range of the milestones you should expect.

Whether your child is 8 months old, 18 months old, 3 years old, or beyond, you can find out what he should be doing physically, cognitively, in terms of speech, and more. For example, is he able to feed himself, drink out of an open cup, and calm himself down within the age range provided on the site? Or is he having frequent tantrums and problem behaviors because he doesn't understand the world around him?

If you find that your 2-year-old is reaching all the milestones for a typical 18-month-old but not yet the 2-year-old milestones, it could be that he's just a bit delayed. But if he's 2 and doesn't have some of the skills of a typical 12-month-old or 15-month-old yet, it may be more indicative of a serious delay.

If your child already goes to daycare or preschool, talk to his teachers to see if he's falling behind in the classroom. A teacher can give you input as to how he's responding to the group and whether he's behind in important milestones.

If there are any delays between what your child is doing and the developmental milestones, definitely continue with the strategies within the book, and take the actions recommended.

## Step Three: Begin your own assessment.

As soon as one of the moms in our online community noticed some regression in her son's skills, she immediately got a professional early assessment and put her child on three evaluation waiting lists. Yes, I know I've said it's an emergency, but don't go into a panic and try to do everything at once. As I said, the first step is to finish reading this book. If your child is only slightly delayed, the techniques you'll read about here may be enough. If you rush to see professionals before you know what your child truly needs, and they are "old school" with their assessment strategies, you might receive some of the poor advice I've already mentioned.

We'll talk more in Chapter 4 and beyond about how to handle your child's early assessment needs and begin to get appropriate professionals in place. But immediately, I recommend that you complete the Modified Checklist for Autism in Toddlers (M-CHAT). This screening tool is frequently used by pediatricians at the 18-month-old and/or 24-month-old "well check" visit, but you can download and complete the M-CHAT for free at m-chat .org. It's valid for children 16 months to 30 months old and can be completed in just a few minutes.

The M-CHAT consists of 23 questions, such as: Does your child point with his index finger to show you things? Does your child pretend or play make-believe? Does he make eye contact with you? Does your child enjoy bouncing on your knees and singing songs? Is your child or was your child delayed with walking? Many of the questions require a simple yes or no answer, but it's an excellent starting point that will help you determine the best course of action.

## TAKING BACK YOUR POWER AS A PARENT

As you begin to observe your child or assess what to do next in regard to his treatment, my goal is for you to be empowered to help him make progress. Before we get to the early assessment information, however, I want to discuss an even more urgent topic: how to keep your child safe.

# CHAPTER 3

# Keep Your Child Safe at Home, at School, and in the Community

Chino was not quite three years old the day his mother went into his room to get him dressed, as always. But when she opened the dresser drawers, she found them empty.

"Where are Chino's clothes?" she asked his dad.

"I don't know. I didn't touch them."

His parents soon discovered that Chino had managed to open his second-floor bedroom window on his own and throw all of his clothes out onto the roof. Then he even closed the window by himself.

Five-year-old Sam, who had been diagnosed with moderate-to-severe autism, went to New York City on vacation with his parents. As they were waiting in line to board the ferry for a visit to the Statue of Liberty, Sam's father's belt set off the metal detectors. He had to remove it in order to go through, and in the confusion, Sam darted out of sight of both his parents. Only seconds passed before they realized he was gone, but panic set in. This was unfamiliar territory to them. Was he in the street somewhere? Had he gotten on the ferry without them? Luckily, they were able to find Sam within about 10 minutes. But this was the longest 10 minutes of their lives, and the outcome could have been much different.

When my son Lucas was small and we'd go to gatherings like a family barbecue, I would sometimes ask a relative to watch him while I went to the bathroom. They would, of course, say, "sure." But inevitably, by the time I came back from the bathroom, he had wandered off, and they weren't aware he was gone.

They were watching Lucas as they would a typically developing child, but the truth is that children with autism or developmental delays require much more attention. While you can trust most three- or four-year-olds to stay on the sidewalk with you, a child with major language delays won't understand the concepts of street, curb, stop sign—or why they shouldn't go into traffic. Many of our kids with delays simply don't have the ability to understand danger or assess if a situation is safe. And this will remain true into adulthood for some with moderate-to-severe autism.

I'm not telling you these stories to frighten you. But I know from a survey I conducted with my community that parents of children with autism or delays rated safety as their biggest challenge. That's why this chapter comes before most of the rest of the book. I know that keeping your child safe is your number one priority.

First of all, as parents, we have to assess our children realistically and not assume they understand what a typical child would at the same chronological age. They may, for example, be able to speak but not fully grasp the meaning of what they're repeating back to you or what you're saying to them. Ensuring their safety requires that they have good language comprehension, not just the ability to speak. Many young children also have attention issues, and some are very impulsive. Because of their delays, they don't always have the ability to think before they act.

Lucas, for example, had no sense of danger when he was young. When he was two and three, he would wander away from home or when we'd take him to the mall. Once, my husband had Lucas in a double stroller with Spencer at the mall. Lucas hopped out of the stroller, ran out the door of the store, and got lost for 20 minutes.

Even for kids who have higher language abilities and are less impulsive, there are safety concerns with identifying danger. As Lucas aged, we might have been able to teach him to dial 9-1-1, but we couldn't teach him to assess if there was an emergency that merited a call to 9-1-1.

Even though there are specific risks involved with raising a child with delays or autism, the good news is that there are many strategies to keep your child out of harm's way—in your home, in school or care facility settings, and in your community. Let's start with the home.

## SAFETY AT HOME

"You need a fence," my neighbor said to me one day after watching me try to prevent two-year-old Lucas (who was not diagnosed) and one-year-old Spencer (who went from crawling to running in the span of two months) from darting outside our yard.

"Oh, no," I said, "my husband doesn't want a fence." But I was running myself ragged every day as my sons ran in opposite directions.

"You need a fence!" my neighbor repeated emphatically.

She was so right. I was losing my mind. So we gave in and got a fence, and it was a game-changer. A fence is just one of the many things you can and should consider adding to increase safety.

It's important to bear in mind that as your child grows, his physical abilities may increase more rapidly than his ability to assess dangerous situations. For example, he'll get taller and be able to reach doorknobs and cabinets. His physical dexterity will also increase so that he might be able to open bottles or jars. He could drag a chair and use it to get to a high cabinet.

Below are some safeguards I recommend you consider putting in place in your home.

- **Install locks and alarms.** One study showed that almost half of children with autism wander into unsafe situations,[1] so you may need physical barriers to prevent them from leaving. To keep your child from exiting the house, install locks that can't be opened from the inside or alarms/bells that will go off every time the door opens.

- **Put doorknob covers and hook-and-eye locks on doors within the home.** Install doorknob covers that your child can't manipulate. These are helpful within your house to prevent him from entering the bathroom and kitchen where he could access soaps, knives, or other seemingly safe utensils. Some children with autism eat inedible things such as shampoo or small objects (a condition called pica). One of my clients used to go into his brother's bedroom and eat inedible objects. His parents installed hook-and-eye locks high on the doors to make sure he couldn't enter rooms without supervision.

- **Install cabinet and drawer locks.** Place locks on all cabinets and drawers from which your child could reach anything dangerous (bearing in mind the possibility that he might stand on a chair). He might pull down heavy things on top of him or reach medications, sharp tools, or toxic cleaning supplies. None of these items should be accessible. I also recommend buying nontoxic cleaning supplies. They are less dangerous for the whole family and also better for the environment.

- **Put covers on electrical outlets.** Making outlets inaccessible is preferable to constantly saying, "Stop touching the outlet." That kind of negative reaction will make it harder to get your child to respond to positive reinforcement. By making it impossible for him to touch the outlets, you can stay as positive with him as possible.

- **Notify your neighbors and local police department that your child has autism or delays.** If your neighbors and police officers are aware that your child might leave the home, they will keep an eye out for him and be ready to help.

- **Get a medical alert bracelet and/or GPS band.** A medical alert bracelet can be helpful to identify your child if he gets lost, and GPS systems with a wristband or ankle bracelet can track him so that you can find him if he wanders. These safeguards are dependent on someone finding him before anything happens, however, so it's even more important to prevent him from getting outside in the first place.

- **Get window locks.** As the opening story about Chino made clear, windows also need to be made safer. Even a child under the age of three may surprise you and open windows. I've heard of children who have climbed out windows onto the roof. Of course, ensure that the child can't manipulate whatever locks you put in place but also make sure that the windows throughout your home can be opened in case of a fire.

- **Have a fire safety plan.** In addition to making sure windows can be opened by adults and older children without delays, it's also important to have a fire safety plan and practice that plan with your entire family. Working smoke and carbon monoxide detectors, fire extinguishers, and fire safety ladders that can be stored underneath beds are important for all families, especially if you have a child with autism.

- **Place gates at stairs.** If your child is likely to take the stairs up or down when you're asleep or not around, you might need to place gates at the bottom and/or tops of steps.

- **Secure furniture to the wall.** All children are at risk of pulling heavy furniture on top of them, but once a typical child has reached a certain age, he'll probably understand not to do that. A child with a language delay or autism may not understand the risk. So I recommend bolting to the wall any furniture that could possibly be turned over. There are anti-tipping cables that you can purchase to prevent these furniture mishaps.

- **Cook carefully.** Whenever Lucas was in the kitchen as I cooked, I used the burners on the back of the stove. You may also want to put covers on the burners and monitor your child around all heat sources, including grills and fireplaces.

- **Install an anti-scald device.** While your young child should never be able to turn on hot water while alone, you can give yourself additional peace of mind by either turning down the maximum temperature on your water heater or installing an anti-scald device that prevents the temperature of the water from reaching a dangerous level. Once Lucas reached the age where he could shower on his own, we installed one of these in the bathroom so that the water would never become too hot.

Besides these suggestions, walk around your home and look for anything that could be a hazard. Even light bulbs can be a problem for some kids who might touch them and get burned. I know that as parents, we hate to anticipate the worst, but it really is better to be safe than sorry.

## SAFETY AT SCHOOL OR DAYCARE FACILITIES

Kelsey's older son, Brentley, was diagnosed with autism at two. Before Kelsey found my Turn Autism Around online program, she drove an hour each way three times per week so that he could attend an ABA clinic, where he sometimes got out of the facility and bolted into the street. As a single mom, Kelsey had her hands full because she not only had to worry about keeping Brentley safe, but she also had another son, Lincoln, who was only one year old and starting to show signs of autism, too.

You may have read stories in the news about kids like Brentley who dart into the street and older kids with autism who wander from school and end up missing. It's every parent's worst nightmare. Unfortunately, some schools and care facilities aren't set up to deal with children who have the tendency to bolt. If your child is at risk of running away, you may need to ensure that he has one-on-one support from an adult while at school, daycare, or any other facility where you aren't there to watch him. In addition to teaching language skills, a trained one-on-one aide can also keep your child engaged and safe by providing prompting, reinforcement, and guidance for playing with other kids.

It helps to assess the school or facility for risks. Here are some questions to ask as you review the areas where your child may be throughout the day:

- Bolts and locks are just as important in schools and other facilities as they are at home. But schools have different regulations to follow so gates and bolts are oftentimes prohibited. If it isn't possible to use a gate or the classroom door, can a staff member always be positioned between the door and your child?

- Are windows left open, or are they easy to open without a staff person's knowledge?

- Are there items in the room that could be hazardous to your child if he gets hold of them before an adult realizes it?

- Are bathrooms safe, and will your child be supervised when there?

- Will your child be on a playground, and is that area fenced in? Are there hazards within the playground, and how will your child be supervised while there?

- If your child rides a school bus, will he be supervised on the bus and when transitioning from the bus to the school building?

If any of these are issues that might affect your child, you need to make sure there's enough support in place to prevent danger. I know this can feel daunting, but these are important safety problems to solve.

## AUTISM AND WATER

Sadly, drowning is the number one cause of death of children with autism. For some reason, they seem to be attracted to water, which was certainly true for Lucas. I know someone whose six-year-old son wandered away from his home and drowned when a neighbor's gate was ajar. He got into their yard and into their pool while no one was around. The mom of this boy has since become an advocate for how to prevent other parents from going through the same thing.

For example, if your child has only experienced the water with floaties, teach him how to swim without floaties as early as possible. This way, if he ever ends up in a pool or body of water unsupervised, he'll have the skills to swim. He needs to know how to get to the side of the pool and needs to learn how to put his face in the water. If possible, get one-on-one instruction from a professional to teach him how to be safe in the water, how to float on his back, and eventually, how to swim. If you have a swimming pool, put a gate around it. If your neighbors have swimming pools or hot tubs, ask them to stay vigilant about keeping their gates locked.

Close supervision of young children around all water sources, not just pools, is also important. If your child has more significant impairments like Lucas does, these safety measures are essential regardless of his age. In addition to receptive language delays, children with autism are also at higher risk for seizures, so even a seizure in a bathtub or a child-size small pool can be dangerous.

Again, I know these stories are frightening, but if you take precautions, there's no reason your child with autism shouldn't be able to enjoy supervised time in water.

# SAFETY IN THE COMMUNITY

Brentley frequently darted away from Kelsey and didn't respond when she called his name or shouted "stop" or "come back." So she had to either carry Brentley in a backpack and Lincoln in the front, or carry the baby and use a harness and leash to keep Brentley with her when they were in the community. Like

Kelsey, some parents feel like they have no choice and resort to using backpack leashes that their young children can't remove or oversize strollers, even for older children.

The good news for Kelsey and Brentley is that after she implemented the Turn Autism Around strategies, she was able to phase out the backpack harness. It took a few months of work, but Brentley started responding to his name and stopped darting away. Sometimes, it takes trial and error to discover what command your child will respond to. One of my clients has a son who wouldn't respond to "stop," but he did come to her when she said, "Give me your hand."

Parents often ask me, "How can I teach my child street safety? How can I teach him when to stop and when to go? How can I teach him to avoid strangers?" You can try to teach him these things, but be realistic about what he can truly understand. Remember that he may be able to repeat what you've taught him without comprehending it. You may find that it simply isn't possible for your child to understand these kinds of dangers yet.

Experts say typically developing kids shouldn't be allowed to cross the street alone until they're 10 years old. That's average, of course. Some typical kids may still not have the decision-making skills to do that at 10.

However, even with young children who are functioning very much like toddlers, you can certainly try to teach them general safety awareness, especially to stop at streets, to be aware of cars and parking lots, to not dart off, and to hold the adult's hand. But still, you need to stay close. Not only do they not have the decision-making abilities to cross the street, but they may be impulsive and dart out into traffic.

Also, as soon as possible, once your child is talking, you can and should teach your child his name, address, and telephone number in case he gets lost. This information should be available on a medical alert bracelet or GPS tracker, too.

Here's another helpful tip: When you're out with your child, have edible reinforcements or something else fun with you that will keep your child busy and entertained as much as possible.

(Reinforcements/reinforcers are items that *reinforce* and increase "good" behavior. In this case, having reinforcers readily available and delivering them frequently should increase the chances that your child will stay with you.) This will help to prevent him from becoming distracted and running away from you. Then when he stays by your side, praise him for it!

For opportunities to play outdoors, look for parks and playgrounds in your area that are fenced in. It may be worth driving a bit out of your way to access such a park where your child can't run outside of the area.

When you travel to a new environment such as on vacation, you have to be particularly vigilant since you probably won't be able to have the same safeguards in place as you do at home. We once rented a beach house, and Lucas got out. Since he's attracted to water, we were very scared, but luckily, we found him on the sidewalk near the house.

If your child has a GPS tracker band, be sure to expand its range before you travel so that it will work wherever you are. I know of a family whose child wandered off on a large cruise ship, and they had to search for him on several decks in a panic.

## SAFETY PRECAUTIONS WILL PUT YOUR MIND AT EASE

It may feel as though all the safeguards you need to put in place will make your home like Fort Knox, but you'll be happy you did everything necessary to keep your child as safe as possible. Then you can turn your attention to improving the *quality* of your child's life.

In the next chapter, you'll learn how to quickly assess your child's strengths and needs in as little as 10 minutes so that you can figure out the best starting point.

# CHAPTER 4

# An Easy Assessment to Figure Out Your Starting Point

"Mary, I haven't been trained. How can I possibly do an assessment of my child?" I hear this question from parents all the time.

Not only *can* you assess your child, but you *must*. Experts, teachers, and therapists will come and go, but you will always be the best teacher and advocate for your child. No one sees him more than you do, and no one will ever know him better. Your assessment will matter even if he's currently on a waiting list for a professional assessment. Even if he's already had speech and behavioral evaluations and is receiving treatment, it will matter. Even if he previously had numerous assessments from experts, with or without a clear diagnosis, it will matter.

With your own regular assessments, you will alleviate a problem I see frequently—poor collaboration between home, school, and therapists. It will allow you to be sure that the interventions you undertake at home are complementary to the therapies your child receives from others—and vice versa. Only you can make sure that everyone is on the same page.

It's especially important to start interventions if your child is wait-listed for an assessment or therapy. You *cannot* afford to lose that time. This was certainly true for Kelsey and her older son, Brentley, whom we discussed in the last chapter. After being on a waiting list for a year, he was finally diagnosed with autism at the age of two. Then he was on another waiting list for three months before his therapy was to start. Meanwhile, he was unsafe, banging his head on hard surfaces up to 100 times a day. As you already learned, he frequently darted into the street and toward water. Kelsey needed to stop these dangerous behaviors as quickly as possible, so assessing him, planning, and starting her own interventions were imperative.

Shortly after Kelsey implemented the TAA approach with Brentley, she started to be concerned about her baby, Lincoln, right after he turned one. Even though his signs were very different from Brentley's, this time, Kelsey had the tools and knew what to do to assess Lincoln herself and start implementing a home program without professional help.

She had to wait a year to get Lincoln diagnosed. He received his diagnosis at 25 months, the same age as Brentley. While Lincoln did qualify for autism treatment, by the time he was evaluated and diagnosed, his language was all caught up, thanks to Kelsey springing into action.

> With the help of my simple Turn Autism Around assessment form, you'll be able to see the whole picture quickly, regardless of your training or experience level. You can print out or access the electronic copy of this assessment form and all forms in the book at
>
> **TurnAutismAround.com.**

I know this is hard to believe, but it should only take about 10 minutes to finish this assessment. Afterward, you may identify concerning issues that are hiding beneath the surface. For example, a child with no ability to speak will almost always have eating issues and difficulty with play and imitation. If they can't ask for what they want, they're likely to have problem behaviors, too.

Since issues like these are so often related, it's vital to get that big picture vantage point quickly. People often ask questions about problem behaviors like, "How do I get my child to stop _____?" Fill in the blank with anything from hitting other kids to banging his head on the floor to refusing to eat certain foods. But as tempting as it is to focus on a specific problem behavior, it will almost always backfire without an assessment to give you a full understanding of the child's abilities, language, feeding issues, sleeping, toileting, self-care skills, and more.

You'll then have the confidence to continue assessing your child's progress and creating new plans as his skills grow and develop. I recommend completing this assessment form and creating a new plan on a regular basis (which will be covered in the next chapter).

As you work on your assessment, you'll need to review typical milestones discussed in Chapter 2 so that you can compare your child's abilities to what is expected for his age. This will help you have realistic expectations. You don't want to inadvertently expect a two-year-old with developmental delays to be able to do what a typically developing two-year-old can't yet do. I have seen this happen even with professionals who focus on teaching skills that are not developmentally appropriate and way too advanced. That's a recipe for frustration on everyone's part, and it's wasted time for your child. Remember: You have to start working with your child not based on his chronological age, but on where he actually is in his development. He may be 4 years old, for example, but have few language skills and be functioning at only an 18-month-old level for expressive language, while having severe tantrums during eating or potty training. Your assessment will help you understand the importance of working on language skills first, and your plan might include placing skills like potty training on hold for a few months.

# THE ASSESSMENT FORM

At the top of the form, you'll see that it asks you for the date, your name (as the person completing the form, whether parent or professional), and the child's name, age, and date of birth. Since you'll complete the form every few months, it's important to always finish this top portion so that you have an accurate chronological record of your child's development.

# MEDICAL INFORMATION

This short section allows you to list your child's diagnosis if he has one yet. You may currently be on a waiting list for an autism evaluation, or you may already have reams of paper documenting multiple evaluations. Simply write down the most important information in this section, including whether your child is currently going to preschool or daycare, receiving therapies or special services, taking medication, suffering from allergies, sticking to dietary restrictions, or experiencing safety issues, such as wandering or vulnerability to strangers, traffic, and/or water (as you learned about in Chapter 3).

# SELF-CARE

In this portion, quickly assess whether your child can feed himself, and briefly note the textures and types of foods he will eat. Does he use bottles, pacifiers, straws, and utensils?

Include a line about sleeping patterns and issues, if any, as well as a short note about potty training or difficulties. We'll cover how to do more in-depth assessments on feeding, sleeping, and potty training in later chapters.

When most parents think about delays and signs of autism, they think about speech delays, lack of eye contact, and maybe some odd behaviors or excessive tantrums. But a big part of assessing a child's developmental level and his strengths and needs involves looking at self-care skills, including independence with

# Turn Autism Around Assessment Form
## by Dr. Mary Barbera

Date of completion _____
Person completing _____
Child's name _____
Age _____ yrs _____ months
Date of birth _____

### Medical information
Diagnosis (if applicable/known) _____

_____
Age of diagnosis _____ yrs _____ months
Does your child currently go to school
and/or receive any therapies or special
services? Yes ☐ No ☐ If yes, please list
schedule and location of services (home,
school, clinic) _____

_____
Current medication _____
Allergies _____
Special diet/restrictions _____

_____
Safety awareness concerns (check all that
apply): Wandering ☐ Strangers ☐
Traffic ☐ Water ☐

### Self-Care
Describe eating and drinking patterns.
Please indicate if child can feed self, what
texture/types of foods he/she eats. Also
list issues with bottles, pacifier, utensils,
straws, etc. _____

_____
Describe sleeping patterns/issues _____

Describe potty/toileting issues _____

_____
Describe grooming/dressing issues
(brushing teeth, washing hands, etc.)____

_____

### Speaking/Expressive Language
Does your child ever use any words?
Yes ☐ No ☐ If yes, please describe the
amount of words and give examples of
what he/she says _____

_____
If no, does your child babble? Yes ☐ No ☐
If yes, please list sounds you have heard:

_____

### Requesting/Manding
Can your child ask for things he/she wants
with words? Cookie, juice, ball, push me?
Yes ☐ No ☐ If yes, please list the items/
activities your child requests with words:

_____
_____

If no, how does your child let you know
what he/she wants. Circle the options that
apply: gestures/pointing/pulling an adult/
sign language/pictures/crying/grabbing

### Labeling/Tacting
Can your child label things in a book or
on flashcards? If so, please estimate the
number of things your child can label and
give examples _____

_____
_____

### Verbal Imitation/Echoics
Can your child imitate words you say?
Single words Yes ☐ No ☐
Phrases? Yes ☐ No ☐

Does your child say things he/she has
memorized from movies or things he/she
has heard you say in the past? Yes ☐ No ☐
If yes, please describe: _____

_____
_____

### Answering Questions/Intraverbals
Can your child fill in the blanks to songs?
For example, if you sing "Twinkle, Twinkle
Little _____," will your child say "star"?
Yes ☐ No ☐

Please list songs that your child fills in
words or phrases to: _____

Will your child fill in the blanks to fun
and/or functional phrases such as filling
in "Pooh" when he/she hears "Winnie the
_____"? Will he/she answer "bed" when
he/she hears "You sleep in a _____"?
Yes ☐ No ☐

Will your child answer WH questions
(with no picture or visual clues)? For
example, if you say "What flies in the sky?"
will your child answer "bird" or "plane"?
Will he/she name at least three animals or
colors if you ask him/her to? Yes ☐ No ☐

### Listening/Receptive Language
Does your child respond to his/her name
when you call it? Circle the frequency that
applies: Almost always/Usually/
Sometimes/Almost never

If you tell your child to get his/her shoes
or pick up his/her cup, does he/she follow

your direction without gestures? Circle
the frequency that applies: Almost always/
Usually/Sometimes/Almost never

If you tell your child to clap his/her hands
or stand up will he/she do it without
gestures? Circle the frequency that applies:
Almost always/Usually/Sometimes/
Almost never

Will your child touch his/her body parts,
for example, if you say "Touch your nose?"
Yes ☐ No ☐ If yes, please list the body
parts he/she will touch without any gestures from you: _____

_____

### Imitation
Will your child copy your actions with
toys if you tell him/her "Do this"? For
example, if you take a car and roll it back
and forth and tell your child "Do this" will
your child copy you? Yes ☐ No ☐
Will your child copy motor movements
such as clap hands or stomp feet if you do
it and say "Do this"? Yes ☐ No ☐

### Visual/Matching
Will your child match identical objects to
objects, pictures to pictures, and pictures
to objects if you tell him/her to "match"?
Yes ☐ No ☐ Unsure ☐
Will your child complete sign-appropriate
puzzles? Yes ☐ No ☐ Unsure ☐

### Social/Play Concerns
Circle all that apply: eye contact/greeting/
playing with toys/sharing/pretend play/
response to name

### Problem Behavior
Is your child currently able to sit at a table
or on the floor and do simple tasks with an
adult? Yes ☐ No ☐ Unsure ☐

Please list any problem behaviors (crying,
inattention, hitting, biting, lining up toys,
stimming/scripting, etc.) and estimate the
frequency (100x/day, 10x/wk, 80% of the
day, one time per day): _____

_____
_____
_____
_____
_____

dressing and washing hands. So on the assessment form, you'll record if your child can dress himself at all, such as pull on his pants, and wash his hands or brush his teeth. (Obviously, keep in mind that if your child is 12 to 18 months old, some of these skills are not yet expected for typically developing toddlers either.)

Dr. Mark Sundberg, Ph.D., BCBA-D, who wrote the foreword for my first book, *The Verbal Behavior Approach*, is the author of a much more in-depth assessment and curriculum called the Verbal Behavior Milestones Assessment and Placement Program (VB-MAPP). This assessment was published in 2008 and is used and recommended by many professionals in the ABA field. In addition to the main VB-MAPP assessment (which we will cover briefly in Chapter 9), Dr. Sundberg also created a few supplements to the VB-MAPP and has graciously allowed me to reprint sections of his four-part self-care checklist within this book to help you better assess your child and complete the TAA assessment form. The best thing about the VB-MAPP and the self-care checklists is that Dr. Sundberg used developmental milestone charts to carefully align everything to match how typically developing children acquire and learn new skills.

You'll see parts of Dr. Sundberg's self-care checklist here and in later chapters. (The link for the entire self-care checklist is also available at TurnAutismAround.com.)

This four-part checklist includes dressing, grooming, feeding, and toileting in developmental sequences that children usually acquire by 18 months, 30 months, and 48 months of age. The most helpful aspect of this list, however, is that it shows you the order that the skills are generally acquired. Completing the checklist will allow you to complete a more detailed assessment of critical self-care skills.

So for instance, using a portion of Sundberg's dressing checklist found here, you can easily see the prerequisites of a skill. If your child can't yet take his socks and shoes off or pull down his pants, which are all 18-month skills, it isn't time to start teaching him to put on shoes or put on pants, which are skills that come a year later for most typically developing kids.

DRESSING – BY ABOUT 18 MONTHS

___ Pulls a hat off
___ Pulls socks off
___ Pulls mittens off
___ Pulls shoes off (may need help with laces, buckles and velcro straps)
___ Pulls coat off (may need assistance unbuttoning and unzipping)
___ Pulls pants down (may need assistance unbuttoning and unzipping)
___ Pulls pants up (but may need help getting pants over a diaper, and with buttoning, snapping and zipping)

DRESSING – BY ABOUT 30 MONTHS

___ Unties shoe laces
___ Unbuttons front buttons
___ Unsnaps
___ Fastens and unfastens velcro
___ Unzips front zippers (smaller zippers may be difficult)
___ Removes shirt (tight shirts may require assistance)
___ Removes pants or skirts (may need help unzipping and unbuttoning)
___ Puts on shoes (needs help discriminating right from left and tying)
___ Puts on pants (may need help zipping and buttoning up)
___ Adjusts clothing
___ Matches own socks
___ Matches own shoes
___ Puts dirty clothes in a hamper

# SPEAKING/EXPRESSIVE LANGUAGE

Now that you've completed the medical and self-care portions of the TAA assessment form, assessing language is next. Language skills make up the bulk of the assessment form. This is because communication is so vital.

Here, you will note if your child uses any words, and if so, write down examples of some of the words he frequently says. If he doesn't use words, does he babble? If so, describe some of the sounds you've heard.

# REQUESTING/MANDING

*Manding* is a term that means "to make a request." It was coined by behavioral psychologist Dr. B. F. Skinner in his 1957 book, *Verbal Behavior*. Many young children with autism or delays struggle to request what they want. Manding is a very important skill because there's something in it for the child—there's personal motivation. For example, as adults, we're motivated to get a paycheck, so we work. When kids can't ask for what they want, there will inevitably be problem behaviors, and it will be difficult to move on to the other language skills if your child isn't manding. There is little point in trying to get him to label objects or answer questions if he can't at first request what he wants.

Can he ask for what he wants using words like *cookie* or *water*? If yes, list the items he frequently requests.

If your child doesn't currently mand verbally, does he let you know what he wants through other means? Circle on the form the ways your child asks for things, such as by using gestures or pointing.

## LABELING/TACTING

*Tacting* is another term coined by Skinner, which refers to labeling. This is sometimes a more advanced skill than manding, but some kids with autism or speech delays can tact or label some things before they can ask for what they want or need. Can your child label real objects and pictures in a book or on flashcards? It can be helpful to show different combinations of objects and pictures of the same item to make sure he can identify a real banana, for example, as well as a picture of one. On the form, write down the words your child can label, or if he has dozens or hundreds of words, estimate the number of items he can label and note a few examples.

## VERBAL IMITATION/ECHOICS

Echoing is an imitation skill, and once a child starts to echo, it often opens up the floodgates to language. If you ask your child to "Say 'ball,'" will he say "ball"? If you say "banana," whether or not you're holding one up, will he say "banana"? Does he repeat phrases he has memorized from movies or phrases you've said in the past? If your child does this, it's called "delayed echolalia." While "scripting" lines from movies can be a red flag for autism, if your child is talking, it's a good thing. But if he won't echo words and phrases spontaneously or during teaching, his language may not grow. Many young children with autism or severe language delays don't echo spontaneously, but you'll learn the secrets to get your child to echo later in this book. So don't get distressed as you note your child's echoic skills on the assessment form.

## ANSWERING QUESTIONS/INTRAVERBALS

Intraverbals refer to the ability to answer questions or fill in blanks to songs or phrases. Can your child name colors or animals when you ask? Can he say "star" when you sing "Twinkle, Twinkle, Little _____" or fill in "bed" when you say, "You sleep in a _____"?

Also, assess whether your child can fill in the blanks to phrases like "ready, set, GO" and can answer simple questions with no picture or visual clues, such as "What flies in the sky?"

You'll learn more about intraverbal language in the advanced language chapter, but for now, it's important to document if your child has any intraverbal abilities.

## LISTENING/RECEPTIVE LANGUAGE

Manding, tacting, echoing, and intraverbals are all examples of verbal behavior or *expressive* language skills. *Receptive* skills refer to how well your child understands what others say to him and how well he follows directions without any visual prompts. But it's complex to assess these skills, so parents often make mistakes during the process.

Before Lucas was diagnosed, I inadvertently assessed his ability to touch body parts by always touching each part on my own body as I said or sang the "Head, Shoulders, Knees, and Toes" song slowly. When I touched my head and sang "head," Lucas found it easy to touch his own head because (1) I always sang the parts in the same order, and (2) I modeled touching my own head. He was just imitating me and learned the order of the song without actually learning the parts of the body. When he was asked to point to any body part without the song and in a random order or without anyone pointing to their own body, he was unable to do it.

These are the kinds of things that trip up professionals, let alone parents, if they don't know to watch for them.

So in this portion of the form, you'll assess your child's ability to comprehend language without any prompts. Does he respond to his name, for example? If so, how often? Is he able to follow simple directions such as asking him to stand up or clap his hands without a demonstration of the action from you? Will he touch his body parts if you ask without showing him? A good way to make sure you assess receptive language correctly is to sit on your hands while you say, "Touch nose," or "Get your coat."

## IMITATION

Imitation is one of the most important skills to assess, as typically developing children learn most language and social skills through imitation. Can your child copy what you do when you ask, such as roll a car back and forth after you show him? If you clap your hands and say "do this," will he also clap? Does your child copy you or his siblings spontaneously?

## VISUAL/MATCHING SKILLS

Can your child match identical objects to objects, pictures to pictures, and pictures to objects? Is he able to complete puzzles that are appropriate for his age? To assess matching skills, you can put three different pictures or objects on the table and hold one matching picture or object up as you say "match." Simultaneously hand the picture or object to your child. He might need a little help to get the idea that you want him to put the matching picture on top or put the objects that match next to each other. Even if your child can do jigsaw puzzles, test him on inset puzzles since you'll use these simpler puzzles while teaching to enhance language skills.

## SOCIAL AND PLAY CONCERNS

Social and play skills are usually a big concern for parents of young kids with delays. In Chapter 7, we'll look more deeply into assessing and teaching these critical skills, but for now, just circle your concerns. Are you worried about eye contact? Does your child fail to respond to his name and show no interest in waving "hi" and "bye" to people? Do you have concerns about his ability to play appropriately with toys, to share, and to pretend play?

## PROBLEM BEHAVIORS

We tend to think of problem behaviors strictly as big outbursts, acts of aggression, or self-injurious behaviors, but they include anything that's disruptive. For example, I worked with a boy who asked over and over to go to a particular restaurant. It was difficult to distract him from this. Another client liked to put straws in bottles and line up toys for hours. This is what we call "self-stimulatory behavior" or "stimming," and it's often an issue with kids who have little or no language skills. While these aren't tantrums, they still might be problem behaviors. So when you assess this area, it's important to consider a wide range of behaviors that get in the way of your child's learning.

Can he sit at a table and do simple tasks with you or another adult? When you run a vacuum, does he scream? When it's time for a bath, or when he wants candy at the grocery store, what does he do?

When you answer these questions, be more specific than just saying, "throws a tantrum." Does he scream, flop on the floor, hit, kick, punch, or bite when he's told no or needs to complete a hard or non-preferred task? Does he cover his ears when there are loud noises? Write down the exact behaviors you observe because these will evolve as he learns more and more, and your records will help you keep track of his progress.

## RECORDING VIDEOS

In addition to completing the one-page assessment, I recommend that you record two short (1-minute) videos before proceeding with your plan.

- Video 1 should be of your child alone, doing something without anyone engaging with him.

- Video 2 should be of you and your child engaging (or you trying to engage him) in some learning activity.

Also, if your child has any problem behaviors, or you're concerned that the behaviors you're seeing might be related to a medical issue such as seizures or tics, I recommend recording a short video or two to document his baseline (his beginning status before interventions) of any concerning behavior. Then share it with professionals. Similarly, if your child has any open wounds or marks caused by a behavior, take a picture as a baseline with the date recorded and share it with your child's doctor.

IMPORTANT NOTE: As you learned in Chapter 3, your first priority is keeping your child safe. So don't record anything if it can't be done safely and discreetly.

## BASELINE LANGUAGE SAMPLE

In addition to the TAA assessment and the two videos, there is one more assessment that you should do before proceeding with planning. This is a baseline language sample. You can do this by setting a timer for 10, 15, 30, or even 60 minutes. During this time, you'll record the date, time, and all sounds or words you hear your child say. If you do more than one language sample, you might begin to see patterns of more talking in the morning or during time outside.

Here are examples of baseline language data for three different children. Please don't feel discouraged if your child is like Child 1, who isn't talking or babbling yet. This is just a snapshot, and since you're reading this book, you and your child will learn and make progress.

---

Name: <u>Child 1</u>   DOB: <u>09/15/XX</u>   Age ___ yrs ___ mo
1 hour – 9/15/XX, 12–1PM in family room

No words or sounds heard.

---

Name: <u>Child 2</u>   DOB <u>03/20/XX</u>   Age ___ yrs ___ mo
15 minutes – 06/16/XX, 8:30–8:45 AM in family room

Ba ba ba, while reaching for bottle
Ooo
Ahh
Mama when shown picture of Mom

---

Name: <u>Child 3</u>   DOB <u>05/14/XX</u>   Age ___ yrs ___ mo
30 minutes – 9/17/XX, 2:00–2:30 PM outside

Words heard:
Slide
Push me
I want swing
Go, with prompting of "ready, set, ____ "
Open
Mommy go in

---

I know you may be tempted to skip this part and move ahead to get to the "good stuff" where you learn how to implement strategies. I understand that you're anxious to see progress. But I urge you to complete the Turn Autism Around assessment form, the two 1-minute videos, and at least one short language sample before proceeding. In addition to using these assessments to build your plan, which you'll learn next, you'll also have a permanent record of your child as he is today.

I suggest you record these short videos and language sample on a regular basis as you update the assessment and the planning form. Keep the completed forms in a binder and/or in a safe digital file. These will help you in so many ways, and you'll be glad to have them as your child starts to make progress!

## BUILDING YOUR CONFIDENCE

I know you may feel nervous about assessing your child— worried that you won't do it right. But just begin. You'll learn as you go, and you'll become more confident about your assessments as you apply the strategies and see results. No matter what, you're putting your child in a position to have less stressful and more productive days ahead.

In the next chapter, you'll learn how to use the TAA assessment to create a plan so that you know which skills to work on first.

# CHAPTER 5

# Gather Materials and Make a Plan

Cody's mom, Jenna, was a teacher, so when he showed delays early on, she knew that it was important to get early intervention services in place. Before the age of one, there were big gaps in his development, especially in motor functioning. Jenna was most concerned about the fact that he didn't roll over, sit up, or pull himself to standing on time. The multidisciplinary evaluation team found Cody was delayed in several areas, so he qualified for a physical therapist (PT), an occupational therapist (OT), a speech and language pathologist (SLP), and a developmental teacher who each came to work with him at home or within his daycare setting for one hour per week.

But Cody wasn't making great gains with these services and was falling further behind, so he was evaluated by a developmental pediatrician around 18 months of age who (much to his parents' surprise) diagnosed him with autism and recommended ABA. But Jenna, who was pregnant with her second child, didn't know where to go for ABA, so she continued with the same services and plan. When Cody returned to the doctor six months later, the gap had grown larger, and the doctor was adamant that ABA was needed. So even though Cody had four hours per week of early intervention services and many goals in place since the age of one, the gap continued to grow.

Cody is an example of a child with delays in multiple areas who had a plan and services in place but wasn't making much progress until ABA was started. The majority of parents who have a young child who is delayed don't know how to navigate the system and help their child catch up. Often, one parent is in denial (like I was), and the waiting lists for even a simple speech evaluation can be long.

Because Lucas didn't have any obvious physical delays like Cody, no one evaluated all areas of Lucas's development until he was almost three. Even though we had speech goals in place and weekly therapy to address his language deficits, he fell further behind, and the differences in his development from typical kids were undeniable.

If the assessment of your child and his current delays have left you feeling sad, I've been there. But the time to begin to catch up is now.

It's important to be realistic, however. If your 3-year-old hasn't yet met the milestones of a 9-month-old or a 12-month-old, skills like potty training or learning prepositions may need to be put on hold. You wouldn't try to teach him to walk before he has learned to crawl or stand. So you have to begin from his true developmental level and not his chronological age. When you engage professionals, make sure they're also realistic. Sometimes, both parents and professionals select goals that are too difficult, and this can make the situation worse. When Kelsey's son Brentley began learning interventions, he had problem behaviors and couldn't mand or label objects. Yet his therapist tried to immediately work with him on identifying colors. That was far beyond his capabilities.

Similarly, when Lucas began working with a speech therapist at the age of two, he was able to request bubbles, but that's pretty much where his manding ended. The therapist was unaware that his manding abilities needed to improve before he could move on to other expressive language skills. So she tried to get him to understand the concept of "one" versus "some" versus "all" and tried to teach him the concept of "yes" and "no." But these were advanced skills beyond his abilities. In fact, he didn't manage to acquire those skills until a few years later.

While you may worry that you won't always know which skills to work on first, using the TAA assessment and plan will guide you. It's important to share this information with the professionals in your child's life and to begin to more actively advocate for what he needs. Remember: you need to become the captain of the ship, making sure that your child's time is used to maximize his results.

If you haven't finished the one-page assessment yet, the two short videos, and the language sample from Chapter 4, please go back and do that before proceeding. With those assessments complete, I'll show you in this chapter how to make sure your child's goals and plan are individualized to his needs. You'll complete a planning form and discover how to create an inviting learning environment for teaching. I'll also provide a list of the simple items you'll need to gather to start the process. You'll learn about pairing and reinforcement as well, which are crucial elements of success for both you and your little one.

## PLANNING FORM: STRENGTHS AND NEEDS

It should take only about 10 minutes to complete the TAA planning form. Start by looking at the first column of the TAA assessment form. If your child has safety concerns, such as wandering or bolting into streets, this will be your first need on the planning form. If he eats a variety of foods, put this in the strengths area. Continue on to the middle column, and document your child's strengths and needs in terms of manding, tacting, etc.

You can find a blank planning form at TurnAutismAround .com, and I've included a filled-out planning form here that I used for my former client, Faith. She was diagnosed with autism at age two, but I didn't start working with her until she turned three. From her TAA assessment form when I started, she refused to sit at the learning table, and she couldn't echo or verbally imitate. She also couldn't answer questions, sing songs, or match identical objects. Plus, she flopped on the floor about 10 times per day.

Faith had some important strengths, however, that were noted in her assessment. She was able to request a few of her favorite things when she wanted them (mand) and label objects (tact). She could say about 50 words, could feed herself, and slept through the night. She responded to her name most of the time and sometimes followed directions as long as they were accompanied by gestures.

When her parents completed the TAA planning form, they noted her strengths and her needs. Then they made a simple plan to work on the first skills they wanted to help her develop. You'll note that potty training was also a need on their list, but since Faith had problem behavior (flopping) and language skills that needed to be addressed, it was put on the back burner for a few months.

In Faith's case, there are more strengths than needs, but it's common to have more needs than strengths when you're just getting started with teaching.

Again, I highly recommend getting a binder and a three-hole puncher to keep you organized, starting with the assessment and plan. You will update both every few months as your child progresses. Keeping these forms organized allows you to go back and see exactly how much progress your child has made.

Now, let's create an inviting environment for your child's learning.

## Turn Autism Around Planning Form (Sample)
### by Dr. Mary Barbera

Child's Name: Faith      Date of Birth: 1/5/XX      Date Form Completed: 4/20/XX

Age: 3 years 2 months

| Strengths | Needs |
|---|---|
| • Can say 50 words<br>• Can mand and tact<br>• Feeds herself<br>• Sleeps through the night<br>• Responds to her name most of the time<br>• Follows directions sometimes when accompanied by gestures | • Cannot echo/imitate<br>• Cannot sing songs<br>• Cannot match identical objects<br>• Flops on the ground several times daily<br>• Potty training |

| Plan |
|---|
| • Pair table and materials with reinforcement<br>• Learning time at the table daily<br>• Focus on echoic control and visual matching<br>• Collect data on language and problem behaviors |

## PREPARING YOUR TABLE TIME LEARNING AREA

When we started teaching Lucas, we used our basement as his therapy room, but we needed to make some adjustments. In order to create the best environment for learning, you'll need to identify a space with limited distractions. So it's important to carefully choose the area where you will teach your child new skills at the table. It can be a separate room in your home or the corner of a room, but it's helpful to have a door or gate that you can close, if possible. While you can use your child's bedroom, it's best to avoid it if they have sleep issues.

When selecting the best learning area, you must be able to "sanitize" the teaching area. When I say "sanitize," I don't mean that you need to pull out the bleach wipes or clean. Sanitizing in this case means you need to pick an area where you will be able to remove any objects that could distract your child from the teaching—especially anything he might want, such as toys. So a room filled with toys, books, and lots of clutter is not the best area for teaching, as you'll struggle to prevent your child from leaving the teaching area to find toys or other distracting items. One of the reasons you may need to use a gate or close the door to the table time room, especially in the beginning when you start table time sessions, is to avoid the need to sanitize the whole house.

## THE IMPORTANCE OF TABLE TIME

The focus on table time is one of the key differences between the Turn Autism Around approach and traditional early intervention (EI) programs for toddlers with autism or other developmental delays. I developed a system of pairing specific materials and procedures at the table to increase pro-social or "good" behaviors like sitting, attending, talking, imitating, matching, and following directions. This is not only important for early intervention, but it provides the building blocks to all future learning.

Most EI professionals who are not familiar with my approach recommend "following the child's lead" and doing activities on the floor, which may look more "age appropriate" on the surface. For example, if you're following your child's lead and sitting on the floor as he pulls out a cow from a farm toy, his EI professional might suggest you hold up the cow to see if he might echo you and say "cow." But then your child might get up and run to the window. You might then say, "Oh, look! A tree!" But he might move away from the window without echoing you this time. After that, he could grab a favorite toy or a pacifier and run out of the room as you chase after him.

Before you know it, a half hour has passed, and you, the EI professional, and most importantly, your child have barely made any gains at all. Time is of the essence with children who are delayed, so when you make table time fun and teach in a structured way, you will get many more learning opportunities, and your child will almost always make progress more quickly.

Here's why the Turn Autism Around approach to table time works:

- Selecting a room or a corner of a room for table time—with specific materials that are kept only for table time—allows you to structure learning time for you and your child.

- Having your child sit at a table with you builds joint attention. When he happily sits and eventually requests his favorite items, activities, and your attention, he soon realizes that you are the giver of all the good things and that learning is fun!

- Teaching matching, imitation, labeling, puzzle-building, and most early learner skills are easier with a flat surface. You can also switch activities quickly while your child stays at the table, allowing for a lot more learning opportunities.

- The skills you and your child learn at the table can then transfer to the natural environment so that your child can be learning at bath time, in the playroom, or at the grocery store.

The most important thing to remember about table time is that it needs to be fun! We want our children to run or at least walk eagerly to the table and willingly sit for short learning sessions. You'll learn more in the upcoming chapters about getting your child to love (or at least like) table time.

## GATHERING MATERIALS FOR TEACHING

The materials you'll gather for your short teaching sessions should be kept in a separate bin or closed cabinet that's out of reach so that they're only used when you can engage with your child. Puzzle pieces and parts of toys need to also be well organized in separate bags or containers. If he can play with the items whenever he wants, it will be more difficult to get him to sit still and engage with you during learning time. If your child is very young or engages in mouthing objects (regardless of age), keep all small parts of toys and materials out of reach to avoid any risk of choking.

Essentially, the teaching/learning area should include the table, chairs, teaching materials, and reinforcers we'll discuss in the next section.

I recommend getting a child-size table and at least one child-size chair. You or other adults working with your child can sit on a regular chair, on the floor, or on the sofa with the table pulled near it for teaching time. The size of the small table is important, as your child's feet should be on the floor, not dangling. But he should be free to come and go from the learning table unless there are safety issues.

**HERE IS A CHECKLIST OF BASIC MATERIALS THAT I SUGGEST YOU GATHER FOR YOUR TABLE TIME SESSIONS:**

\_\_ Child-size table and chair(s)

\_\_ Reinforcing items (edibles, a drink, an electronic device, bubbles, etc.)

\_\_ A shoebox with a large slit cut in the top so that it's easy for your child to put flashcards and pictures through it

\_\_ Two identical packs of first word flashcards

\_\_ Two duplicate sets of pictures of family members and favorite items (Mom, Dad, juice, tablet, etc.)

\_\_ Mr. Potato Head, keeping all the parts in a separate clear bag

\_\_ Three or more inset puzzles

\_\_ Simple cause-and-effect toys, such as a hammer and balls, pop-up toys, or toys with parts that can go in or down

\_\_ A first word book and simple books with pictures and up to one sentence per page

\_\_ Two sets of six identical items (toy cars, spoons, cups, bowls, small dolls, etc.)

To make the learning area fun, think about what reinforcements you can use. I usually recommend that you plan for at least two edibles cut into small pieces, one drink, an electronic device, and some of your child's favorite toys and books.

The two packs of first word flashcards and copies of photos of reinforcing items and people will also be used for the shoebox program and other early learner programs like matching, which we'll discuss in Chapter 8.

When you purchase your first word flashcards, try to find cards with realistic pictures that don't include letters or words on the front with the picture. If your flashcards do include text, you may need to modify them a bit. For instance, if a flashcard contains the picture of a cat but also the letter *C*, I recommend covering the letter with a blank label or otherwise removing it. Children with language delays or autism may focus only on the letter.

Besides the preprinted flashcards, print out photographs of your child's reinforcing items like juice, a tablet, and a cookie, as well as pictures of Mommy, Daddy, siblings, pets, and any family members and friends with whom your child has regular contact. Print out duplicates of each photo so that you can also use these same pictures later to teach matching skills.

It's important that the photos you print *only* contain one person or one reinforcing item with no extraneous items. Don't include a photo of your child drinking from his juice cup, your child with his pet, a picture of the whole family of four, or Mom on a bicycle wearing a helmet. This is too much stimuli that can be confusing for your child. Also, make sure the pictures you use are large enough to see clearly with the photo's subject in focus.

Pick books that have simple pictures and few words. You can continue to use other books at bedtime, but keep the books you've chosen for the table with the other table time materials.

You'll learn the actual teaching techniques in the upcoming chapters. I know you're eager to get going, but I want to give you a little time to get your learning area ready and gather the needed supplies before I explain how to use the materials. It's important that you resist the urge to jump ahead to the chapter that corresponds with the skill you want to teach first. For the sake of your child, following my step-by-step system out of order is a mistake you don't want to make.

## PAIRING AND REINFORCEMENT

*Pairing* refers to using things your child likes (including bubbles, snacks, attention, etc.) and delivering these items without any demands. This makes every activity more positive and fun. Pairing is not a one-time thing, though, so if your child resists any task like putting on his shoes, you'll need to focus on pairing or re-pairing the activity to make it easier.

In addition to delivering reinforcing items, you also want to pair all external reinforcement with praise using simple gestures such as smiling and giving a thumbs-up and words or phrases like "That's great!" You can also clap and simply say "Yay!" when your child is successful. In the beginning, you may need to deliver reinforcement *every time* there is the slightest success.

A student came to observe a session I conducted years ago with a toddler, and she couldn't believe the amount of positive reinforcement that was necessary to get the child to participate in the learning. It may feel like I'm recommending an excessive amount of reinforcement, but I assure you it isn't excessive at all. This is how you help your child learn and make the most progress.

Many parents have said to me that they worry that reinforcement is akin to bribery, but there's a distinct difference. Bribery isn't planned; it's a reaction to problem behavior. If your child starts screaming for candy at the grocery store, and you offer him the candy to get him to quiet down, that's bribery. Even if the candy works to settle your child down at the store, it's a short-term change that will cause the problem behavior to worsen over time. Offering candy during a tantrum teaches your child that if he cries, he will get good things. So this bribery in the grocery store only reinforces the problem behavior you don't want, and that behavior will then almost always spill over to bath time, bedtime, and learning time.

Reinforcement, as opposed to bribery, is planned. Good behaviors like sitting, imitating, and talking are reinforced often, which results in long-term positive change. With bribery, the child is actually in charge and gets what he wants. With reinforcement, the adult is in charge of planning and delivering reinforcement when the child is being "good" and exhibiting the behaviors you want to see more often.

So as you plan and start to teach your child, don't hesitate to go overboard with lots of praise and positive reinforcement. It

# Bribery vs. Reinforcement

## Bribery

•Not planned out
•Reactive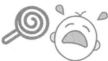
•Follows problem behaviors
•Often involves negotiation
•Behavior worsens, short-term change

## Reinforcement

•Planned out
•Adult led
•Follows good behavior
•Delivered with praise
•Long-term positive changes

won't do any harm as long as you aren't reinforcing crying and other problem behaviors.

Now that you've completed the assessment and plan, and while you're gathering the materials for table time, you're ready to learn a key strategy that you can start today.

# THE SINGLE MOST IMPORTANT PAIRING STRATEGY: USE ONE WORD X3

Over the past two decades, I've found that my "One Word x3 Strategy" is the single most effective pairing method to help increase talking.

When using this strategy, which is central to the Turn Autism Around approach, you'll use single words and say them slowly in an animated way *up to* three times in a row before delivering reinforcement. I say "up to" three times because if your child echoes you after the first or the second time you say the word, you'll want to deliver the reinforcement item immediately. If your child loves bananas, cut the fruit into several pieces. Say "banana, banana, banana" up to three times as you deliver each piece. If he says "banana" or "nana," deliver the piece as quickly as you can. Then when you hold up the next piece a minute or two later, you might wait a few seconds before saying it and delivering it to see if your child will mand for it more spontaneously. Finally, if your child is having problem behaviors or you're losing his interest when you say words three times in a row, you may need to quicken your pace and vary the number of times you repeat the words.

If your child has limited speech or is not talking at all, avoid talking to him in complete sentences, as he may not understand. By saying only single words, you may feel like you're talking to him in a babyish way, but I've found that if you keep your words simple, his comprehension and language abilities will increase more quickly. Also, the number of syllables in a word is more important than the length of the phrases or sentences. So use words with few syllables, especially if your child is completely nonverbal at this point.

If your child wants to be picked up, for example, avoid saying, "Okay, I'll pick you up, Susie," which may sound like garbled nonsense if she has little language comprehension. Instead, say, "up, up, up" right before you lift her. When you open a door, say, "open, open, open!" As you help your child out of his booster seat, say, "down, down, down."

You can use this One Word x3 Strategy throughout the day in every setting even before you formally start table time. It will begin to pair you as the teacher and pair words with reinforcement. It might even start to increase your child's language skills.

However, please don't start table time, use the materials, or place a lot of new demands on your child until you read the next few chapters. Rushing to try to "fix" all your child's deficits and catch him up all at once can backfire.

In the next chapter, you'll learn how to deal with tantrums and other problem behaviors. Please read this chapter even if your child isn't exhibiting any major behavioral issues yet.

# CHAPTER 6

# Stop the Tantrums and Start the Learning

Every child with and without delays will cry and have occasional tantrums, but children with autism or signs of autism, especially those with severe language impairments, tend to have many more problem behaviors. This is because they usually don't understand rules as well as typically developing kids and don't have the ability to use language well enough to get their wants and needs met. So when we tell our children no and keep piling on demands that are not based on their developmental level, they have meltdowns.

Before we dive deeper into how to stop tantrums and other problem behaviors, however, it's important that you've read the previous two chapters and completed the assessments and plan. These are big pieces of the puzzle. Also, even if you think your child doesn't have any big behavior issues, please don't skip this chapter, as I will guide you through addressing all barriers to learning, whether you call them "problem behaviors" or not.

You've read about Kelsey already, but I think her older son Brentley's problem behaviors demonstrate how bad things can get. As I mentioned, it took a year of waiting for the autism diagnosis and then another three months to get Brentley into an autism ABA clinic. During those 15 months before Kelsey learned about my approach, Brentley ran away from her, bolting into streets and toward water so often that she felt the need to use a leash and harness to prevent a catastrophe. In addition to these dangerous behaviors in the community, when Brentley didn't get what he wanted, he screamed, flopped on the floor or ground, and banged his head up to 100 times per day. The behavior analyst at the ABA clinic was so concerned about the self-injurious behavior (SIB) that she even suggested Brentley should wear a helmet to protect his head if he was going to continue to attend sessions.

Kelsey ended up finding my Turn Autism Around online programs right before the helmet suggestion was made. Even though she had waited so long for the diagnosis and professional treatment to start, and insurance was paying for ABA, she realized that going to the clinic was making things worse, not better. The therapists there weren't using the strategies she was learning in my course. Since they were working on colors before Brentley was able to mand for any items or sit and attend to materials for even five minutes at a time, Kelsey felt strongly that the reason for his extreme behaviors was that the demands were too high and the reinforcement was too low.

It was brave of Kelsey to walk away from the professional help that was being paid for through insurance, but she knew she had to do something to start turning things around for her son. Within a few months, Brentley's head banging went from 100 times per day to near zero levels, he learned to love the learning table, and he no longer darted away from his mom and was much safer around water and cars.

Of course, not all kids have huge issues like Brentley. My former client Jack seemed pretty mild-mannered when I first started working with him shortly after he turned two and was diagnosed with autism. He came to the door holding a straw and smiled at me when I entered his home for my first consultation.

His mom and dad reported that Jack was mostly pleasant and had few problem behaviors. But Jack liked straws and loved putting them in clear bottles. He also enjoyed lining things up. He wasn't talking, had very few skills, and was very resistant to sitting at the learning table. It took me six hours over the course of three visits to figure out how to encourage Jack to willingly come to the table to sit!

During the first month of weekly consultations, I learned that Jack also had feeding and selective eating issues. Even the sight of mushy food would cause crying and tantrums, so to try to keep him calm and happy, Jack's parents presented only finger foods that he would accept without crying. While Jack wasn't engaging in aggression or self-injurious behavior (SIB) like Brentley was, his problem behaviors were definitely preventing him from learning language and social skills.

You might not think that extreme picky eating, spending a few hours each day lining up toys, or putting straws in bottles would hurt anything, but they are real problems. During the first few years of life, the brain of your child is being "wired." The best scenario is that every waking hour (~100 hours per week) is spent engaging him to catch up on social and language delays in a positive and fun environment with little to no problem behaviors present.

If your child has tantrums or any other problem behaviors that prevent him from learning new skills, whether they are severe like Brentley's or milder like Jack's, resolving these behaviors must be your first priority. It's simply impossible to teach a child anything while he's having a tantrum, screaming, or crying. You might think that hugging your child to try to calm him down or trying to pick him up and carry him away from a situation is the answer. But these strategies will almost always backfire in the long run. Keep in mind that your child will eventually be too big to pick up and carry (if he isn't already), so it's important to tackle problem behaviors as soon as they appear. The goal is to get any *minor* problem behaviors, such as lining up toys, crying, or whining way down and to get any *major* problem behaviors like hitting, head banging, or flopping to the ground to zero or near zero levels.

In Chapter 4, I explained the importance of figuring out your child's starting point and quickly documenting his behavior problems. In this chapter, you'll learn how to become a detective to determine the *cause* of the behaviors so that you can *prevent* them rather than simply react.

Remember that your child is using the behavior to try to communicate with you. It's natural that your first impulse is to give him a hug, hold him, or give him what he wants to stop the crying or tantrum. While this may work in the short term, it will turn into more severe problem behaviors in the long term. And if you or your partner, your child's grandparents, or his childcare provider think that imposing some kind of discipline is the answer, know that it almost always backfires, too. Keep in mind that any child engaging in a tantrum is already frustrated and upset. Punishments and threats are likely to make the behavior worse.

If a child is crying or having some sort of tantrum, it's no longer a "win-win" situation. You have two choices at that point: to react to or ignore the behaviors, both of which could cause the problem behavior to escalate.

The key is to spend 95 percent of your time on preventing all problem behaviors, so in this chapter you'll learn how to be as proactive and as positive as possible.

Ponder this question: If I offered you $1,000 for your child to have a good day with no problem behaviors, what would you be willing to do to make it happen? You'd probably allow him to do almost anything he wanted. You might let him eat unlimited cookies for dessert or allow him to watch the same videos all day. You wouldn't ask him to do anything he didn't want to do. He wouldn't have to take a bath, wear shoes, or have his meals with the rest of the family. In short, you'd give him free access to reinforcement and few demands.

As counterintuitive as it may seem, this is where you need to start to prevent problem behaviors. You want to give lots of free access to things the child likes, while making as few demands as possible. Of course, no matter how hard you try, it's virtually impossible to make no demands on your child. You can't allow a toddler to eat a whole box of cookies or let a four-year-old go to preschool without shoes. But in general, you want to catch a child when he is "being good" and be the "spoiling grandmother" by giving him lots of reinforcement in the absence of problem behaviors throughout the day. Limit saying no and avoid non-preferred and difficult tasks as much as you can until you learn more about how to teach him to communicate and get major problem behaviors near zero levels.

# FUNCTIONS OF BEHAVIOR

In my first book, *The Verbal Behavior Approach*, as well as in my online programs, I discuss the four functions of behavior. One important point that I don't think I make enough is that all behavior, not just problem behavior, occurs due to one or more of the four functions.

All "good" or pro-social behavior like talking and imitation, as well as tantrums and other problem behaviors, occurs because of a history of:

1.  gaining access to items, attention, and information we need or want;

2.  avoiding difficult or undesired tasks;

3.  stimulating our minds when nothing else is happening; and

4.  alleviating pain or discomfort.

The first function is to get something desirable. This is the reason children engage in "good" behavior like saying "train" or "milk" or engage in "bad" behavior like crying. Both behaviors—talking or crying—would get your attention and could lead to a child gaining access to a favorite item. This function is often seen when children have to wait or are told no when they request something. Brentley, for example, asked for juice, and when his mom told him no, he began crying and flopping on the floor.

The second function is to get out of doing something. This is the reason why kids argue, negotiate, or have tantrums. Let's say your child doesn't want to take a bath. If he has a decent amount of language, he might argue and beg in a demanding voice for 30 more minutes of TV before his bath. But if he's not talking or has limited access to language, he might whine and cry. You might decide you can delay the bath by 30 minutes or that he can do without a bath that night. This may lead to your child learning that he can get out of his bath (and other non-preferred tasks) if he protests by arguing, whining, or crying.

The third function or reason is to get sensory stimulation, which can result in good or bad behavior. All our leisure activities give us sensory input. But young children with delays rarely have the ability to engage in age-appropriate play, so they tend to have problem behaviors when they aren't occupied and given lots of positive reinforcement. One of my former clients, Christopher, was so under-stimulated by his well-meaning babysitter that he banged the back of his head for hours every day just because he liked the way it felt. Other types of self-stimulatory problem behaviors are rocking, making noises, repetitively lining things up, or *verbal stimming*, in which the child repeats certain sounds, words, or phrases without understanding their meaning.

The fourth function is often forgotten and is physical or medical in nature. A child or adult who is fully conversational can understand why they need to take medicine or have an IV placed. They can describe pain and ask for medicine to relieve it. Children with autism or severe language delays can't communicate in this way, so they might bite their hand or become aggressive when in pain or under stress. Biting their hand might help alleviate pain, such as a headache. This may seem strange, but you may have seen old movies in which someone performs surgery before anesthesia existed. The patient is given a towel to bite on to help alleviate the pain of the surgery in the other part of the body. So biting is a well-known way to diminish pain.

If your child exhibits self-injurious behavior (SIB), such as head banging or biting himself, seek out both medical and behavioral professionals right away to assess the situation and help your child. While I'm trying to simplify this issue in this chapter, reducing severe problem behavior is actually quite complex. You will need professionals to recommend measures to protect your child, you, and everyone around him while you work on alleviating the behavior. And even if a medical problem can't be found immediately, keep looking. While you do that, also lower the demands, and provide more reinforcement while your child isn't having problem behaviors.

While you don't have to keep data about functions, it can be helpful to understand which function(s) are leading to your child's behaviors. Keep in mind, too, that the same behavior might have more than one function. You may find, for example, that most of the time, your child resorts to tantrums to get out of particular activities he dislikes, but other times, he goes into a tantrum because he simply wants attention or because you said no to a request.

In many situations, all our behaviors occur because of more than one function. This is especially true during transitioning from a highly preferred activity to something that's hard, new, or scary. An example of this is a child crying when we tell him "all done computer" (access to an item he loves) and then right away say "time to get a bath" (a difficult/non-preferred task). But don't worry—we'll discuss strategies to deal with transition issues later in this chapter.

## ASSESSMENT OF PROBLEM BEHAVIORS USING ABC DATA

Hopefully, you can see that the "why" of problem behaviors has nothing to do with autism or delays. You can use this information to help any child (or adult) decrease problem behaviors.

Also, regardless of the function or functions of behavior, my approach focuses on teaching you how to spend 95 percent of your time preventing problem behavior. The preventative strategies in this chapter are designed to get your child responding, learning, and feeling generally happier. In almost all cases, working on the good behaviors you want will cause the problem behaviors to decrease and sometimes fade away completely.

The key to learning how to prevent and handle any problem behavior is to uncover the pattern that has led to that behavior. Professional behavior analysts use what's called "ABC data," which stands for *antecedent, behavior,* and *consequence.* I'm going to show you how you can use this tool, too.

The trigger that occurs right before the behavior is called the *antecedent.* Some of these are out of your control, such as the ringing of a fire alarm that frightens your child. The majority of the time, however, the antecedent is that you've told your child no or demanded something of him that he doesn't want to do. This is true of typically developing kids, too. But as I mentioned, children with autism or language delays usually have a reduced ability to understand rules or consequences and to communicate to you what they like and dislike.

Antecedents might be your requests that your child put on shoes, take a bath, or go to the car. When my client Annie was called to the kitchen table to eat, she would scream. My client Faith flopped on the floor when her mother told her to put on her shoes because she either struggled to put them on or didn't want to go where they were headed. I worked with a boy named Jacob who became triggered whenever we tried to transition him from the playground to walking the four blocks home. Jacob would cry and sometimes escalate to self-injurious behavior like hitting his head with his hands or on hard surfaces.

The *behavior* part of the ABC data, of course, is what behavior the child exhibits in response to the antecedent. Does the tantrum involve flopping on the floor, crying, screaming, hitting his head with his fist, or harming someone else? In some children, it may start with crying and whining. In general, if children don't get what they want by exhibiting mild problem behaviors, they might escalate to flopping on the ground, followed by banging their head or becoming aggressive toward a sibling.

As you write down the antecedent and behavior data, it's vital to be specific about the behavior, describing it in detail. For example, writing "he melts down" isn't enough. Instead, you'll need to document what "melting down" looks like. Does his meltdown include flopping, screaming, hitting you, or biting his sister? How long does the behavior go on? Does the length of the tantrum vary depending on the circumstances? If your child screams, it can be helpful to note the volume and how long the screams continue. If he gets "anxious," what does that look like for him? Does he pace around the room? Does he put his head down on the table or start to breathe more rapidly? You can't actually "see" anxiety, but you can see and count the behaviors that your child exhibits when he's anxious.

The location of the behavior and the time of day it occurs are also important because behaviors may occur in the same place or around the same time every day. These patterns can help you detect difficult activities, places, or time periods for your child. Maybe your antecedent and behavior data will show that your child tends to have issues before lunch or only at nap time, which will help you focus on preventative strategies. Does this behavior happen only in certain settings but never or rarely in others? Do the behaviors tend to happen when a particular person is around? This is the kind of specificity you want to strive for in your data because it will give you the clues you need for your detective work.

The *consequence* is the last part of the ABC formula. This is simply what happens right after the problem behavior occurs. Some consequences occur on their own. A loud plane flying overhead will pass, and the loud alarm from a smoke detector will eventually stop. But most problem behaviors we see in kids are "turned off" by something an adult does. So when you think about a common behavior you see, I want you to think about the usual triggers and what you do to stop the problem behaviors, if anything. If your child flops on the floor, do you usually walk away? Do you pick him up?

The consequences will probably vary depending on the circumstances. If you have nowhere to go, you might ignore the flopping, but if you have to get to an appointment, you will probably do something to stop it. If this behavior happens in the presence of your spouse, at daycare, or at school, what are the consequences then? Responding in different ways to the same behavior is almost always reinforcing, which means the behavior will continue in the future and influence how your child will react the next time. For example, let's say you tell your child to put on his coat to walk to the bus stop to get his older brother. When he hears this demand (antecedent), he cries and flops on the floor (behavior). Since you're in a rush and don't want your child to become more upset, you decide to drive to the bus stop and tell him he can get into the car without his coat. To sweeten the deal and get him off the floor, you also tell him he can bring his favorite toy in the car. In the short term, this might make sense, but trust me, your child is learning. The next time he doesn't want to do something (whether that's putting on his coat, taking a bath, or trying a new food), he's likely to scream and flop on the floor because that behavior gets results.

From this example, you can easily see how ABC data can help you figure out how to prevent problem behaviors. The following is a simple form you can use to record your behavioral data based on ABC. (Find blank ABC forms at TurnAutismAround.com.)

## ABC (Antecedent, Behavior, Consequence) Chart

| Date/Time | Activity | Antecedent | Behavior | Consequence |
|---|---|---|---|---|
| When the behavior occurred | What activity was going on when the behavior occurred | What happened right before the behavior that may have triggered it | What the behavior looked like | What happened after the behavior or as a result of the behavior |
| Example 1: Jan. 8, XX 10:10 A.M. | Grocery checkout line—saw candy | Reached for candy and was told no | Screamed and dropped to floor | Gave him candy |
| Example 2: Jan. 10, XX 5:00 P.M. | Dinnertime | Called to table to eat | Cried and said no | Let him eat in family room |

# JAN

| SUN | MON | TUE | WED | THU | FRI | SAT |
|---|---|---|---|---|---|---|
| | 01<br>7:30 am<br>Headache<br>Ibuprofen given | 02<br>Allergy shot | 03 | 04 | 05 | 06 |
| 07<br>Late bedtime: 10<br>pm | 08 | 09 | 10<br>4 am woke up<br>crying / SIB<br>SIB - Ibuprofen | 11 | 12 | 13<br>Late bedtime:<br>11:30 pm |
| 14 | 15 | 16<br>2 pm, slight<br>agitation | 17 | 18<br>Dr. M appt. | 19 | 20 |
| 21 | 22<br>Dr. H appt.<br>Sinus Infection<br>Antibiotic Day 1 | 23<br>Antibx Day 2 | 24<br>Antibx Day 3 | 25<br>Antibx Day 4 | 26<br>Antibx Day 5 | 27 |
| 28 | 29 | 30 | 31 | | | |

# THE CALENDAR SYSTEM

Many children exhibit low-level, minor problem behaviors every day, and engage in more severe problem behaviors much less frequently, like once a week or even once a month. Lucas didn't have severe problem behaviors until he was around six, when he started displaying SIB (hitting his head with his hand) and aggression. I remember thinking he hadn't bitten anyone since the age of two, so I was very concerned when he bit me and his brother in the same week at the age of six. Around the same time, he also developed sudden-onset vocal and motor tics and was eventually diagnosed by an allergy and immunologist with pediatric auto-immune neuropsychiatric syndrome (PANS). Luckily, we determined that Lucas's sudden severe problem behaviors were caused by this medical condition and found through trial and error that antibiotics not only got rid of his tics, but also made his SIB and aggression go down to near zero levels.

It was during this time that I developed my calendar system to help me keep track of Lucas's medical issues and problem behaviors. Eventually, most of my clients started to use the same system.

Using Lucas's calendar as an example, in addition to writing down any major problem behaviors like his SIB at 4 A.M. on January 10, I'd also recommend using your child's calendar to note any medications, supplements, or dietary changes, as well as allergy shots, doctors' appointments, and medical treatments. Children with autism are sometimes very sensitive to medications, and their reactions may manifest in tantrums or other unusual behaviors.

Too often, even medical professionals dismiss problem behaviors as a symptom of autism or delays when the issue could actually be physical pain or some other medical problem. It might be as simple as a headache. With Lucas, for example, my calendar data over the years helped me figure out that headaches and problem behaviors tended to come up for him when he was due for an allergy shot. If you think your child's potty or sleep issues might be causing problem behaviors, you can use the calendar system to track those problems, which will be covered later in the book.

While I only use a digital calendar for my personal and business schedule, I use a physical paper calendar just for Lucas's medical and behavioral data. In addition to allowing any members of Lucas's team to document problem behaviors on his calendar, we're able to bring it to every medical appointment to look for trends and adjust medication. I strongly believe that this calendar system is the reason we've managed to improve Lucas's health and reduce major problem behaviors to near zero levels.

So as you gather all your data, be sure to analyze it and look for patterns, including how frequently both minor and major problem behaviors happen. This information will help you determine what to do about the behavior and create a customized plan that will keep everyone in his life in sync. Consistency among everyone who takes care of him—your spouse, your parents, a babysitter, a teacher, a speech therapist, a behavior analyst—will help a great deal.

Unless your child exhibits a severe problem behavior that is causing harm and requires immediate professional help, I recommend keeping data for at least two or three days before creating your plan. Then focus on preventative strategies. While you need to have some reactive tools in your arsenal for the occasions when problem behaviors still happen, your main goal should be preventing the behaviors from happening at all.

## YOUR PLAN AND INTERVENTIONS: PREVENTATIVE STRATEGIES

Your general one-page TAA plan most likely contains your desires to increase your child's language and learning skills and to reduce problem behaviors. The good news is that a happy and engaged child will have fewer behavioral issues. As I've said, the vast majority of your time—95 percent—should be spent *preventing* problem behaviors by engaging your child in preferred activities as much as possible throughout the day, setting up routines, and scheduling reinforcing activities. Then ease in demands on him gradually.

While engaging a child during all his waking hours is ideal, it's nearly impossible without help. If your child has a diagnosis, and you live in the U.S., all 50 states now mandate that insurance companies cover ABA services. So you may want to explore this. With or without a diagnosis, you will need help keeping your child busy. Think about other resources and people who may be able to lend a hand. You may want to enlist the help of grandparents, older siblings, paid babysitters, or even church volunteers who can learn how to help keep your child safely engaged. I know that without Lucas's ABA therapists, as well as my parents and paid babysitters, I would have been much more stressed, especially in the early years.

You learned in the previous chapter that sanitizing the environment, especially for learning time at the table, is important, but you'll also need to think about how to "pair up" many activities throughout the day as you use denser reinforcement. Avoid structuring the morning and then leaving your child with no engagement in the afternoon (or vice versa). The period without engagement is when problem behaviors are likely to occur. So if you need to do the laundry or take a phone call, set up your child to play with safe toys or watch a favorite video.

Remember: if a problem behavior occurs, it's almost always because the demands are too high and the reinforcement is too low. As a parent, it's your job to figure out which demands are too hard or stressful for your child. In the beginning, demands need to be so small that they're barely identifiable as demands. Very gradually increase them as you keep reinforcement and prevention of problem behaviors front of mind.

How do you simplify a demand? Let's say you want your child to say "hi." The truth is that you can't pull words out of him, but you can simplify this demand by giving the direction to *wave* "hi," which is usually an easier task that can be gently prompted as you demonstrate waving.

If your child struggles to complete the task you've requested, feel free to help him. For example, you can help him put a card into a slot in the shoebox or help him put the blocks away if he doesn't respond to your request to do it. Don't give a demand that you aren't willing to help him complete, and try to make sure your demands are doable for him.

While you can't eliminate all demands on children, you want to be the "spoiling grandmother" when the child is engaging in good behavior. Yes, I said *spoiling*. Remember that positive reinforcement is what works! Use an excited, animated voice as you say "Good!" or "Yay!" or "You did it!" every time he complies. Clap, smile, or give a thumbs up or a high five if your child enjoys it. Think about how much you enjoy it when someone praises you and creates a positive environment. Children need it even more. The goal is to provide five to eight positives for every demand or negative word. If you find yourself saying "no" or "stop" a lot, try to add some positives and strive for a better positive to negative ratio.

Besides praise and positive gestures, consider using the following external reinforcers, especially at the learning table but also to prevent issues during other activities: small pieces of edibles, sips of a favorite beverage, short clips of a favorite video that you can play for 10 to 30 seconds at a time on an electronic device, bubbles, and preferred toys.

Some people don't like the idea of using external reinforcers, especially food and electronics. But children with delays usually need them in addition to praise to increase their motivation to learn. You need to reduce the problem behaviors, especially the major ones, so that you can teach your child and give him a chance at having a better life. If, for some reason, you can't or don't want to use food or electronics, don't stress about it. But it's important that you have a handful of reinforcers and not rely on just one.

Children with delays are often very picky about their likes and dislikes, whether foods or non-foods. So make a list of your child's favorite foods, drinks, videos, audio recordings, toys, and activities. Include movements he enjoys that would usually happen away from the learning table, such as bouncing on an exercise ball or jumping on a trampoline. You can test certain reinforcers by placing them on a table and observing which ones your child selects. It can be helpful to put the reinforcers on your list in order of his preference.

Of course, at some point, your child may have his fill of even his favorite thing, whether that's candy or a video. Plus, his preferences will change as he grows. This means that assessing your child's reinforcers will be ever-changing and not a once-and-done task. There's usually some trial and error involved for you as a parent. It's another reason why your data will be helpful.

You can also prevent tantrums if you think about how to make each activity more fun, whether it's a teaching activity or a task you need your child to complete for daily living, such as taking a bath or eating a meal. Your child might not like the bathtub, or the water temperature may be too cold or hot. You could experiment with the temperature to discover what he likes and could try to re-pair the bathtub with foamy soap or alphabet letters that he can stick to the sides. Maybe practice getting him in the bath fully clothed without water in order to desensitize him to the tub. Perhaps it's just the hair washing part that he dislikes. Attending to what your child likes and dislikes will help you discover the real issues and find a way to prevent the meltdowns.

We'll discuss more about desensitization of bath time, doctor visits, and haircuts in Chapter 13. But for now, please know that pairing and re-pairing activities is a big part of preventing problem behaviors.

## USING REACTIVE STRATEGIES TO "TURN OFF" TANTRUMS

While you will focus 95 percent of your time on prevention, you'll also need to know what to do with the 5 percent of your time when you can't prevent a tantrum. Remember: if your child is crying or having a tantrum, he isn't learning, and once you see crying or tantrums, it's no longer a "win-win" situation.

To "turn off" the tantrums when your child is whining, crying, grabbing, or flopping because he wants an item, I recommend the "Sh, Label, and Give" Procedure, which I developed based on the work of Dr. Vincent Carbone. You can use this for any child with minimal language or even for typically developing infants and young children to help reinforce good behaviors rather than crying or whining.

- Tell your child to be quiet and stop crying by giving the "sh" sign with your index finger over your lips— or ignore the behavior (if it's safe) until he calms down on his own.

- After he's calm for at least three seconds (count silently), label the item one to three times, such as "candy" or "candy, candy, candy," and give the child the item.

These are the most important things to remember when using the Sh, Label, and Give Procedure: Don't give him the item during problem behaviors. It's very important that you get at least three seconds of quiet before saying the item name and delivering it. Don't explain why your child can't have the item. Don't give him other choices. And as long as he's crying or flopping, don't promise that he can have the item later.

If you give in and do any of these things, you'll provide positive reinforcement for the problem behaviors, and the tantrums will increase, not decrease! Also, if you're using reactive procedures many times throughout the day, you'll need to focus more on prevention.

## SHOULD YOU USE TIME-OUT AND
## OTHER PUNISHMENTS?

A punishment is a reprimand or something that's added or taken away, which reduces a behavior. Time-outs and other punishments are often overused for children with and without autism, and I don't recommend them. For one thing, some punishments, such as spanking or using restraints, can be seen as abusive, unethical, or even illegal. Also, decades of research show that all children and adults learn best in environments that are positive not punitive. Even mild punishments like yelling or verbal reprimands can cause your child to withdraw and avoid you. This is the opposite of what you need in order to get him to engage positively with you.

Hitting your child back when he hits you is *never* recommended. Hitting or spanking not only models undesirable behavior and can be considered abusive, but it's also likely to increase or worsen aggression in your child.

What about a time-out? With my two sons, I rarely used this procedure—even before I was a behavior analyst. And I now feel strongly that a time-out should be avoided in almost every case. It simply doesn't work most of the time because it's a reactive procedure rather than a preventative strategy. During standard time-out procedures for 2 to 10 minutes, the child is taken to an area where more or different problem behaviors could occur. While in the time-out, he doesn't learn why his behavior was unacceptable or what he needs to do differently in order to get the reinforcement he wants.

Also, some children may enjoy time-outs, especially if it means they no longer have to do something they don't want to do. This means you might inadvertently reinforce the problem behavior. While most parents and even professionals believe that a time-out is a punishment that will reduce problem behaviors, it often serves as a reinforcer that only makes the problem behaviors increase.

# INTERVENTIONS TO EASE TRANSITIONS

Every child you'll read about in this book has a hard time transitioning from highly preferred activities to non-preferred activities. But honestly, don't we all? Nobody likes transitioning from what they enjoy to what they dislike.

Imagine you're at the beach on a beautiful sunny day enjoying a cold drink and reading a great book. On a scale of 1 to 10, with 10 as the most reinforcing activity, you would probably rate being at the beach a 10. Then without warning, I abruptly approach you and say, "All done with the beach. It's time to load heavy boxes into a truck." Would you like this? Probably not. You might start arguing or slamming your chair onto the sand. You might even refuse to leave.

So the key to easing transitions for your child is to avoid asking him to transition from a 10 (a highly preferred activity) to a 2 (a non-preferred activity). If he's watching a video or playing, and you tell him it's time to go to bed or clean up his toys, this request might elicit a tantrum because he has to transition to an activity he doesn't prefer.

In addition to the preventative and reactive strategies discussed throughout this chapter, here are five ways to ease transitions:

1. **Dangle the carrot (the reinforcement) before the problem behavior occurs.** When my son was little, he loved to be in the ocean for hours. In order to prevent any behavioral issues, I would offer him something else he loved (like pizza) to get him to come out of the water. But it's important to offer the reinforcement *before* you make the demand for the transition. Don't wait until after the problem behavior occurs in reaction to the demand. I would say, "Lucas, time for pizza! Let's get out and dry off."

2. **Don't physically move your child from one location to another.** I wouldn't even think about physically dragging you off the beach to help me load heavy boxes onto a truck. Don't do it with your child (even if he's small enough to carry) unless his safety is at immediate risk.

3. **Whenever possible, offer choices.** In the beach example, if I told you I needed help with heavy boxes, then asking when would be a good time for you to transition would likely lead you to be more cooperative. You might suggest we load the boxes after you finish your drink or as soon as you're done reading the chapter in your book. We make a lot of choices throughout the day, especially when faced with unpleasant tasks. So plan to give your child as many choices as possible before transitions and before any problem behavior begins.

4. **Sandwich harder activities between two preferred activities, and consider using schedules and timers.** It's important that all non-preferred activities are spread out throughout the day and placed between reinforcing activities. Sandwich harder activities between fun, reinforcing ones.

5. **Make sure your learning table is paired with plenty of reinforcement, and try not to use the word *work*.** In my experience, the word *work* is used early and often, especially with kids with delays and it is often paired with hard demands and limited fun. So over the years, I've dropped using the word *work* altogether with young children and would recommend you do the same! Instead of saying "it's time to work," try calling it "learning time," "mommy time," or simply "table time."

## HANG IN THERE

As you implement these problem behavior reduction strategies, be patient with yourself and your child. It may take time to get results, but I've helped enough children to know that these methods are effective. It will be easy to tell if your plan is working because the problem behaviors will decrease or stop. If they don't change or if behaviors worsen, you'll know to reevaluate your data, alter your plan, and seek professional help.

Whatever you do, if your child has a tantrum or exhibits other problem behaviors, remain calm during the episode. Your behavior shouldn't be reactive. If you model appropriate behaviors for your child, he'll become more familiar with what appropriateness looks and feels like. Then later, be the "Monday morning quarterback" who makes a plan to prevent the next problem behavior.

In the next three chapters, you'll learn how to teach language and social skills that will make controlling behavioral issues even easier. In the next chapter, we'll move on to the development of social skills so that your child can more easily interact well with adults and play with other children.

# CHAPTER 7

# Develop Social and Play Skills

When Lucas was two years old, he went to a neighborhood toddler preschool program. This was several months after my husband first mentioned the possibility of autism and I shut him down. We didn't discuss autism at all as we prepared to send Lucas to preschool. We both thought that the environment might help him learn to interact and play with other kids, and we believed the routines and activities would help him develop language.

The toddler class met only two mornings a week, and since Lucas and the other kids were only two years old, the expectations were pretty low with no potty training required. Unlike some of the other children, Lucas had no trouble separating from me when I dropped him off, and he also didn't have any problems with sharing because he didn't care about toys. If another child took a toy out of his hand, he didn't whine or try to get it back.

So in the beginning, because he wasn't causing a fuss, it looked as though he fit in pretty well. But by midyear, the teacher and director of the preschool suggested that we meet to discuss Lucas. While they didn't use the A-word at the meeting, they did say things like, "It looks like he's in his own world most of the time. He's not interacting with the other kids, and he's having a hard time understanding the concepts within circle time. He's not talking as much as the other children."

Their main concern was that Lucas wasn't going to do well when the rest of the class progressed to the three-year-old pre-school classroom. They explained that as children age, the expectations in the older child classes get higher. For example, in the three-year-old classroom, they required all children to be potty trained, and they reduced the ratio of teachers from 2 per 15 kids to just one teacher. They told us that if Lucas was unable to catch up, he wouldn't be able to progress to the three-year-old classroom with his current peers.

We told the preschool staff that we'd already started speech therapy, so we were trying our best to help Lucas catch up. We also pointed out that he was a "young" 2-year-old because he had just turned 2 in July, while some of the other children in his toddler classroom had turned 3 shortly after starting in the fall. So some of the kids were almost a year older than Lucas. They agreed that there was a wide range of "normal" behavior and acknowledged that there were certainly differences between a 2½-year-old and a 3½-year-old in terms of language and development. Nonetheless, it was upsetting to have the director call a meeting with us to highlight our son's delays.

After the meeting, my husband was more convinced than ever that Lucas had autism, and I started to accept that his delays were more serious than I'd thought. Around the same time, our insurance was no longer going to cover private speech therapy at the hospital, so we got an early intervention speech specialist to start working with Lucas in our home. We didn't know to ask for a multidisciplinary evaluation, however, and we didn't tell them we were concerned about autism. So Lucas only received one hour of services from a speech therapist from the age of 2½ to 3, which was another big mistake that further delayed his diagnosis and the intensive ABA treatment I didn't know he needed.

In the end, after Lucas got his diagnosis the day before he turned three in July 1999, we followed the recommendation of the preschool director to have him repeat the toddler class. I later learned that "summer birthday boys" are often held back before entering kindergarten, which is especially true for boys with autism or any type of delay.

Lucas did well as a result of repeating the two-year-old class since the teacher to student ratio was lower, he didn't need to be potty trained, he knew the toddler class routine, and he loved his teacher. He was also able to attend with one of his ABA therapists, which helped a lot in terms of generalizing his skills between home and school.

## HELD BACK OR KICKED OUT OF DAYCARE OR PRESCHOOL

Your child might be older or younger with more or fewer language and social abilities than Lucas had at that time. I've seen many cases where the staff members at daycares or preschools "flag" children if they aren't meeting developmental milestones (such as drinking out of an open cup, waiting in line, or participating in circle time) and aren't ready to move to the next classroom. If you have had this happen (and you've gotten "the talk" like we did) or if your child's quarterly checklists have some concerning scores, don't blame yourself or your child. If someone within a childcare setting or even a concerned family member or friend points out that your child might be delayed, be open to hearing it and start looking more seriously at the typical milestones and red flags described in Chapter 2.

Some children with autism or other developmental delays even get "kicked out" of daycare or preschool settings if their delays are significant and they become disruptive or aggressive toward other children or staff members. Even if your child bites other kids, he's not a "bad" child, and these behaviors indicate that he's struggling and needs more help. This is the time for more assessment and planning, *not* the time for punishment or placing blame on anyone, including your child or yourself.

## DETERMINING IF A DAYCARE, PRESCHOOL, OR ABA PROGRAM IS A GOOD FIT

Your child may already be in a childcare setting or attending a behavioral program, and you're trying to decide if it's the right place for him. Or you may be looking for some of his learning to take place outside the home. If you're determining whether a daycare, preschool program, or specialized ABA clinic/school is a good fit for your child, there are several criteria to keep in mind.

Safety, of course, is first and foremost. Will your child be safe there, considering his particular problem behaviors? Will there be someone there to make sure he doesn't wander, spend all day stimming, or engage in self-injurious behavior?

Observe the children in the school to see if they appear happy. If your child already attends a program, is he happy to go there? Children shouldn't be exhibiting a lot of problem behaviors, especially upon arrival. If they're whining or screaming and don't want to go on the bus or be dropped off, the program probably isn't using the right reinforcement system, and the demands are most likely too high.

Watch the teachers to see if they use negative language like "stop that" a lot. Do they say, "I'm taking the jump rope away if you can't share"? This is a big red flag. Make sure they use positive words and a positive tone as they prevent and react to any problem behaviors. Listen for words and phrases such as, "I like the way you're sharing," "Give me a high five," and "That's so awesome!" As I've said, your child (and all humans) needs five to eight positive statements for every negative one.

Take a look at the classroom schedule. Is there time for specific instruction, or are there large chunks of time engaged in "free play"? Children, especially those with delays, need to have lots of structure, direct teaching, and evidence that they're making progress.

If your child needs one-on-one ABA teaching, speech therapy, or other instruction, is that available at the facility, or will they allow outside support to come to the daycare or preschool to work with your child? How do professionals decide what to work on with each child? Do they introduce demands slowly and focus on pairing new activities? Do they encourage, and are there opportunities for, your child to communicate by manding for what he needs? What information or data do they keep about your child's learning progress and how he functions in the classroom's daily activities? How will this data be shared with you and other members of the team?

Parent and teacher communication at the school or program should be active, transparent, and collaborative. You'll probably need more than communication sheets that show a smiling face for a great day or a frowning face for a tough day. You'll need more detail about what they're working on, about your child's progress, and if he's engaging in any problem behaviors that could signal the need for changes.

In general, you need to find a school or program where staff will keep your child safe and work on the right skills in the correct order, while making sure problem behaviors stay low. This is the only way you'll know if the program is in line with what your child needs based on your most recent assessment and plan.

## EXPOSURE TO TYPICALLY DEVELOPING KIDS IS NOT ENOUGH

Over the past two decades, I've encountered many parents who believe that just exposing their child to other kids will always help and never hurt the situation. But as a behavior analyst, I've found that children who don't understand or use language well may not benefit at all from attending preschool or daycare. In some cases, it can waste time, and time is our children's most important commodity.

For most of our children with delays or autism, just placing them in a classroom with other children won't be enough for them to learn social skills. Most kids with language delays, whether they have an official diagnosis of autism or not, need explicit teaching of these skills first from adults—parents and/or professionals—and only then can they apply those skills to other children. They must learn to parallel play and also pick up some independent play skills before they can benefit from structured group learning.

I started working with my client Adam when he was four. He had some "pop out" words but was basically nonverbal. He was already diagnosed with autism and attending a special needs preschool four days a week. Although he had been in a "Verbal Behavior" type of special needs preschool for a year, I was saddened to learn that he hadn't made any real progress with language, imitation, or matching skills. When I took a closer look while evaluating Adam, it turned out that the special needs preschool staff didn't have the knowledge and experience to program correctly using the VB-MAPP, and they didn't have the capacity to do intensive one-on-one sessions. There were many small group activities like arrival time, snack time, circle time, arts and crafts, and free time. But Adam wasn't using or learning language, and while they had some data collection sheets, the graphs were all flat. For more than a year, he didn't improve at all.

On Adam's one day off during the week, his mother enrolled him in a typically developing daycare setting so that he would be exposed to other children. But since he had no language to communicate with the other kids, he didn't interact with them at all. He had no imitation skills, so he wasn't able to imitate the other kids during circle time or join them during play time. At one point during my evaluation, Adam even licked the wall because he was getting no support or engagement there. But even if he'd had someone working with him one-on-one in that environment, it wouldn't have helped him learn to socialize with the other children. He simply didn't have the language, imitation, and play skills he needed to benefit from that kind of environment.

Some kids don't sit passively like Lucas or lick the wall like Adam. My former client Todd was on the verge of getting kicked out of his four-year-old preschool classroom when I was called in to evaluate the situation. He hadn't been diagnosed with anything, had never received any early intervention services, and on the surface, his language seemed on track. But he had been labeled "bad," and the other kids in the class were afraid of his outbursts. His parents had no idea what to do next, so they paid me to evaluate Todd.

I found deficits in his language and social skills, as well as the absence of positive reinforcement and the overuse of time-outs. I referred Todd to a developmental pediatrician and a speech and language pathologist for a more complete evaluation. He went on to receive a diagnosis of ADHD, and the standardized speech evaluation showed the need for weekly speech therapy.

Luckily, Todd was able to successfully complete the year at preschool with some training of the teachers. By midyear, he was no longer in time-out every day, and he was using his language to communicate. The other kids no longer feared him, and he advanced to the pre-K classroom with a few of his friends to give him an extra year before kindergarten.

If you have other options, I don't recommend putting your child with delays in daycare or preschool most of the day if he isn't yet playing with some toys, imitating, and using language with adults. Of course, if your child needs to be in daycare because of your work schedule or other reasons, you might be able to arrange for early intervention or ABA providers to provide one-on-one teaching there for at least part of the day.

After Lucas's diagnosis, we continued his preschool experience with a second year in the two-year-old classroom because he was used to the routine, liked going, and appeared happy while he was there. He wasn't aggressive or disruptive. It was also only four hours per week, and he was able to attend with a therapist who served as his "shadow." During the two mornings per week, the therapist was also able to see firsthand what skills we needed to work on during his home one-on-one program, and she was able to keep him safe and engaged.

Early social skills include what's called *joint attention*, which involves sharing focus with another person and both looking at an object (like a stuffed animal) or experiencing an activity together. An example of joint attention is when a toddler points to the sky to "show" his mom the airplane flying overhead. He isn't just looking at the sky and pointing; he's trying to get his mom's attention to look at the airplane with him.

Joint attention begins to emerge at around the 9-month-old mark and should be firmly established by 18 months of age. Young children with autism or social language delays often lack joint attention.

Since socialization with adults and other children also requires language, especially once your child reaches toddler age, working on language skills is key if you want your child to become more social. This chapter will get you started in assessing and teaching social and play skills, but the two chapters that follow will help you teach early language skills and more advanced language, which will help with socialization. As you continue reading this chapter, you'll learn that language and social skills are so enmeshed that it's hard to separate them.

## ASSESSMENT OF SOCIAL SKILLS

Two of the biggest social skill mistakes parents make are failing to assess the level of their child's social development and having the same expectations as they would of a typically developing child. This is why it's so important to assess social skills before developing a plan or starting to intervene.

In addition to using typical social and play milestones based on your child's age to determine his true developmental age in this area (which we discussed in Chapter 2), the TAA assessment form has a section to help you assess your child's social abilities and needs. If your child has had any evaluations in the past year or so, I recommend that you also pull out any of those reports, checklists, and evaluations. These may outline your child's standardized assessment scores, strengths, and needs, which may be helpful to you as you work on completing the TAA assessment and plan. I know it might be hard to accept that your child is developmentally delayed by a year or more, but in order to develop the best plan, you need to find your true starting point.

I've summarized some of the key social and play milestones for toddlers and preschoolers below.

# KEY SOCIAL AND PLAY MILESTONES

By 18 months, most toddlers understand "no" and begin to shake their head no and wave. They are aware that people are in the room and when people have entered or left the room. They can sit in a sandbox with other children, although they're more likely to play alone at this stage rather than engage with other children. They will, however, begin to imitate other children and follow them into a playhouse, for example.

Most children without physical or motor delays can manipulate objects and press buttons on a toy by 18 months. They show a variation in play by independently interacting with different toys, such as a ball, blocks, and rings. They are likely to choose new toys rather than only familiar ones when given the opportunity. Children with delays or autism, on the other hand, often repetitively play with just one item.

Most 18-month-old children begin to try movement play, such as jumping, climbing, rocking, swinging, and dancing. They also start to play with pop-up and pulling toys, and they'll begin to dump toys out of containers. Dumping can easily become a problem behavior, though, especially if this behavior is excessive or lingers past the age of two. Lucas used to enjoy repetitively dumping items out of bins and drawers well past the age of three.

Between 18 and 30 months, typically developing children usually begin to hand toys to others in social play. Up until age two, however, they mostly play with toys *beside* other children and just begin to include others in their play. They will start to play pretend, such as feeding a doll, pulling a wagon, brushing their hair, putting a telephone to their ear, and creating traffic jams or accidents with toy cars. They will search for missing parts of a toy, such as a puzzle piece or a bottle for a baby doll. They will begin to use items like a bowl as a drum or turn a box into an imaginary car.

Before the age of two, most children will begin to interact with other children, such as pushing another child in a wagon or holding hands. They will make basic mands toward other kids, such as saying, "push me," "look," or "come on." In turn, they will respond to other kids by looking, following, or pushing a child in a wagon upon request.

During the assessment of social and play skills, it's also a good idea to assess your child at a playground. If he's too small for most of the equipment in the average playground, look for one that's specifically for young toddlers.

In preschool or group situations, children in this age range can usually sit in a group for a few minutes without problem behavior and can transition between activities with minimal reminders. They can respond to verbal directions given to the group, such as, "If you're wearing a red shirt, stand up."

From 30 to 48 months, typical children are expected to show affection for friends and concern for a friend who's crying. They understand the concepts of "mine" and "yours." They begin to participate in imaginary play, such as dressing up, pretending to cook, or having a pretend party with their stuffed animals. They can throw a ball in a basket a few times until they get it to go in, and they understand swinging a bat at a ball. They can work toys with multiple moving parts, such as buttons and levers. They can complete puzzles with three or four pieces and build a tower of six blocks or more.

Most typically developing three- and four-year-old children begin to cooperate with others more, such as holding a bucket while another kid fills it with sand or pretending with other kids at the sand table or while in the toy kitchen area. Language will also begin to develop more and more, as they start to ask and respond to "WH questions" such as "Where are you going?" and "What are you doing?"

Preschoolers should also be able to learn new information and acquire new behaviors in a group setting, such as during circle time. If the teacher reads a book about traffic and red, yellow, and green lights or sings a song about the days of the week, most typically developing children will learn and apply the information immediately without explicit or individualized instruction.

Children between age three and four can usually play for at least 10 minutes on their own without adult involvement or prompting. Of course, children with delays or autism may be stimming rather than actually playing. If you believe this is the case with your child, don't get discouraged. Stimming still means they're exploring and engaging with items. Once you add language and play to their skill set, the sky is the limit as to what they can learn.

## ASSESSMENT

I realize that reading all of those milestones may make you feel overwhelmed, especially if you find that your child is far behind in social skills. But knowing your child's strengths and needs is the first step to turning autism (or delays) around! I've seen many children make great strides in all of these areas when parents take the lead. One of your main long-term objectives is to get your child learning as much as possible in a group setting. So even if your child needs a one-on-one teacher or therapist now to learn the needed skills, keep in mind that eventually, he may be able to learn language and social skills in a group.

In addition to completing the social skill portion of the Turn Autism Around assessment form, completing Dr. Sundberg's self-care checklist, and keeping in mind the typical milestones you've just read, I recommend reviewing the two very short baseline videos.

We discussed these videos in Chapter 4, so now's the time to review them. But just in case you haven't done the videos yet, or if it's been a while and you want to redo them, here's a refresher: both of the videos should be one-minute each—one video of your child playing with toys alone (take this video as discreetly as possible without talking to him) and another in which you'll try to engage with him using toys or play materials at the table or on the floor. Watching these two videos may help you determine his social skills strengths and needs.

Many times, when I've helped to analyze these one-minute baseline videos, I see common themes emerge. In the alone videos, I often see kids repetitively playing with one toy, stacking blocks, or lining up objects. Preschool children with delays might even play with dolls or figurines while they say small scripts/lines from videos.

One four-year-old boy diagnosed with moderate-to-severe autism when he was two lined up pictures of the planets in order and read their names while his mom recorded him. While naming the planets might seem like an advanced skill to some parents and even professionals, it isn't functional. Hours of repetitive play and/or scripting from videos during alone time will almost always widen the social gap and cause children to fall further behind.

The one-minute engagement videos I've analyzed tend to also look similar. Before parents learn how to implement my approach, they often try to get their young child to label letters, numbers, colors, or shapes. The little boy who labeled planets while alone didn't have much functional language, but his mother focused on letter identification during the one-minute table time session. Overfocusing on pre-academic skills and teaching the names of planets is not helpful if your child cannot express their wants and needs and label common objects and people. These functional language skills are needed for a child to develop social language.

## MAKING A PLAN

In Chapter 5, we discussed making a plan and gathering materials to create a learning area with a small table. Now that you have new social skills knowledge, you may want to review and revise your plan. If your child doesn't yet make eye contact, point, or have expressive or receptive language, teaching manners and pretend play won't make sense. Even if he's 3 or 4 years old, you may need to pull out toys for 18-month-olds if that's where his development falls in your assessment. Then you can work on social and play skills both during your table sessions and when you're away from the table throughout the day.

If your child has early intervention or ABA services in place, he'll also have goals. Now that you have your revised assessment and plan in place, you will want to work with the professionals in your child's life to make sure the previously set goals align with your assessment. I've found that standard or cookie-cutter goals just don't work. They must be specific to your child and what he can actually do right now.

# INTERVENTIONS: BASIC SOCIAL SKILLS

As I said earlier, social skills cannot be taught in isolation. My Turn Autism Around approach helps you work on many skills with your child, including social play, language, and problem behaviors all at the same time. But many kids with autism or other developmental delays need systematic intervention based on their assessment and plan to improve socially.

## Teaching Eye Contact

While lack of eye contact is a concern for most parents of young children with autism, you can't teach this skill directly. But it will likely become more natural to him as you continue to teach him other skills. So instead of trying to get him to look at you, position him so that he's facing you rather than the wall during table time. Also, get down to his level whenever possible so that looking at your face will be easier for him. Then hold up reinforcing items, toys, or even pictures of people and things your child likes in front of your face and next to your mouth. Often, I hold an item next to my chin and use an excited voice to try to get the child to look at my face and the item. You can hold up a bottle of bubbles, for example, and say, "Bubbles!" Encourage your child to look toward you and your face, but don't ever try to force eye contact.

## Teaching Pointing

As I mentioned in Chapter 2, failure to point with an index finger by 18 months of age to both request items and get attention can be an early sign of autism or at least a language delay.

There are two types of pointing, however. Making a request for a cookie, for example, is called *imperative* pointing, while pointing at an object or action to gain someone's attention, such as at an airplane, is called *declarative* pointing. Some kids with delays who don't yet point will try to mand or get your attention by grabbing your hand rather than pointing. This is called "hand leading" and can also be a red flag for autism.

Several years ago, when I worked directly with clients like Chino and Max, I discovered through trial and error that teaching kids to point to items isn't that difficult, and I developed a system. If your child can't point yet but is meeting other 18-month milestones, you might want to start teaching him this skill. You can teach pointing throughout the day wherever you are, and once you finish the next chapter and learn more about how to pair the table with high reinforcement, you can also work on pointing during table time. Remember that reinforcers are vital to get your child to want to engage with you, so always work on this skill with strong reinforcement.

Before you begin to teach your child how to point, try to determine his dominant hand. I test this by putting a series of preferred items, such as edibles and drinks, in front of him, midway between both of his hands. Over 10 trials, observe which hand he uses to pick up the items. This isn't foolproof, so observe him in other circumstances too. Then just do the best you can to determine which hand is dominant, and don't worry if he sometimes uses the other hand to point at something. You aren't trying to force him to use one hand or the other; you're simply trying to make it easier for him to learn this skill.

Begin with what we call "touch pointing" with objects that are right in front of the child. At the teaching table, use a book, flashcards, or a tablet. Hold up the item and refer to something specific that's pictured. Let's say you're referring to a duck in the picture. Take your child's dominant hand, and touch it to the item as you say, "Look at the duck!" You don't have to necessarily separate his fingers as you take his hand to point.

Then ask your child to point at it. "Where's the duck?" Until he begins to get it, take his hand again gently and touch it to the picture.

After he has mastered touch pointing, begin working on pointing at objects that are slightly farther away. Stand behind him while he's seated at the table, and hold a book just in front of him. Say, "Let's point to the book!" If he doesn't, hold his arm up, and gently fold down his other fingers with your hand so that the index finger of his dominant hand is pointing at the book. (His thumb doesn't have to be tucked under.)

Then bring the book back down and choose something pictured on the page. Let's say it's an elephant. Hold the book back up at a short distance in front of your child and say, "Let's point to the elephant!" Again, if he doesn't do it on his own, lift his arm by his dominant hand, and gently fold down his fingers except the index finger. For verbal reinforcement, you might want to say, "Awesome!" afterward.

Look for opportunities to point throughout the day, such as pointing at an airplane that flies by while you're playing in the backyard and saying, "Let's point to the airplane!" You might also point toward a sibling and say, "Let's point to your brother!" Even if your child has little language yet, learning to point will help him make choices and communicate what he wants a bit more easily.

## Teaching Simple Greetings

Waving is one of the first skills babies learn, but many children with delays won't acquire this skill without direct teaching, especially if they don't usually notice other people, make eye contact, or have basic imitation skills. So how do you begin to teach them?

Start by thinking about the greeting skill you will teach. Unless your child is already speaking and can echo you, I recommend you work on waving "hi" for now. Always bend down and approach your child at his level. *Don't use his name.* Just say "hi" enthusiastically and wave at him simultaneously. Lift his hand and shake it gently. You will most likely need to repeat this frequently before he begins to wave on his own. You can practice this skill with just the two of you in the room, or if other relatives or friends are available, you can practice greetings with them. Have your husband, another adult, or sibling prepared to practice in another room. Then tell your child, "Let's go say hi to Daddy!" Enter the room, and have Daddy say "hi" and wave. You can gently guide your child's hand to wave as you say "hi" simultaneously.

You can also practice greetings when someone enters your home. Say, "Oh, I hear someone coming!" Get your child to attend to the arrival or departure of this person. Have the person come close to the child at eye level and say "hi!" while waving and *without using the child's name.*

If greeting errors occur, pay attention to whether it's a difficulty with tacting, which would be labeling each person, or an echoic or imitation issue. This means he isn't echoing your words or imitating actions like waving.

Once he masters greeting people with "hi," you can teach him to wave and say "bye," too.

## Teaching Pretend Play

Pretend play is an advanced social skill that requires both expressive and receptive language, which we'll cover more in the next two chapters. Your child may not be ready for this yet, but one of the pretend play activities I recommend is a birthday party. If he doesn't have enough receptive language to understand what you're doing, it could lead to problem behaviors, even if you have strong reinforcers available; but if you feel your child may be ready for it, gather Play-Doh, little plates, teacups, a teapot, and birthday candles. You can say, "Let's make a birthday cake out of Play-Doh!" Then make the cake, put the candles in the Play-Doh, and pretend to blow them out. See if he will imitate you.

It might be fun to have a present for him to unwrap and put an edible reinforcement on his plate. You can show him how to pour pretend tea into the teacups as well. Use your imagination, and see if your child enjoys this. Assess whether he will imitate any of your actions during the activity.

This is an especially helpful exercise, of course, if your child's birthday is coming up or if you're getting ready to take him to a birthday party. You can use the same idea to practice play skills with trains, dolls, or in a toy kitchen. It might be helpful to gather all the materials you need for each play activity in a bin in order to practice different scenarios with the materials. But be careful not to repeat the same activities with the same language over and over, as this will likely lead to rote or unnatural responding and nonfunctional language.

## Advanced Social Skills

I have also seen both parents and professionals try to work on turn-taking (my turn versus your turn) and teach children manners, like saying "please," "thank you," and "I'm sorry" way too early. If your child has difficulty attending to a toy for a few minutes at the teaching table, he won't be able to share with other children, take turns, or understand the concept of being sorry. He simply must master the prerequisite skills before moving on to these more advanced ones.

As I said, social skills, including the ability to play with other children, are advanced and require some pretty complex expressive and receptive language abilities. In the next chapter, you will learn how to teach your child basic language skills, while more advanced language will be covered in Chapter 9.

So be patient, and pay close attention to the order of the milestones/prerequisites so that you don't expect social or language skills that are too advanced too soon. If you help your child master the social skills in the right order without rushing, he will progress faster.

The language skills in the next two chapters are central to my Turn Autism Around approach, so what you're getting ready to learn will be the basis for everything to come.

# CHAPTER 8

# Teach Talking and Following Directions

When Michelle's daughter Elena was diagnosed with autism right before her second birthday, Michelle and her husband were distraught. Elena had started showing signs before she was 18 months old, but her parents received reassurance telling them not to worry, which kept them in denial.

Right before the diagnosis, Elena had a speech therapy evaluation, and even though she was almost 2 years old, the speech testing showed that she was functioning at a 0-to-3-month-old level of language. While she got her daughter the diagnosis relatively quickly, Michelle faced another obstacle when she had to get in a long line for intervention services. She knew she was facing at least three months of being at home alone with her two young daughters—Elena and her newborn sister—without the ABA services she knew Elena desperately needed.

When she began my Turn Autism Around online program, Michelle didn't know how to get her daughter to talk or imitate or how to teach her any of the other skills she needed, but she put one foot in front of the other. After just a week or two of joining, Michelle started making progress with Elena and could tell it was going to be successful. But she had no idea just how successful!

On the first day of the program, Michelle completed the Turn Autism Around assessment and the language sample. Elena's baseline language sample (which you learned about in Chapter 4) included two words—mom and doggy—in the one-hour sample period. Five weeks after she implemented the TAA approach, Elena said more than 180 words in a one-hour language sample. She could even put two words together such as "Mommy's shoes" and "birdie, tweet, tweet." Her cooperation during table time was way up, and her severe tantrums were almost down to zero.

Michelle took her daughter for another speech therapy evaluation when she was 26 months old, and in those short 2 to 3 months when Michelle only implemented what you're reading about in this book, Elena's expressive language age went from a 0-to-3-month-old level to that of a 30-month-old. Yes, she was actually talking like a 30-month-old even though she was only 26 months old. Her social skills were a little behind, still at 20 months, but what a turnaround she'd made with language in a very short period of time with no professional help and her mother as her only therapist.

I tell you this story so that you can see what's possible when you implement the strategies you are learning. But know that each child starts at a different point with a unique set of strengths and needs. Some children like Elena make rapid progress, while others need more time and patience. Whatever the age of your child and whatever his delays, you can make progress and help him get to the next level. This isn't the time to get discouraged or give up!

In this chapter, you're going to learn how to increase language and communication skills in young children who have very little or no language abilities (like Elena did when she started). Even if your child is already saying some words or talking in phrases, do not skip this chapter since it's so important to learn how to engage with him and get him excited to learn language from you.

# HOW BABIES LEARN LANGUAGE

Before I entered the autism world, I never realized how complicated it can be to teach language to children with delays. It still amazes me that typically developing toddlers learn language so easily. It's truly remarkable how quickly they pick up sounds and words and start understanding language. Most babies start babbling when they are just a few months old and experiment with what their voices can do, saying, "baba," "dada," and "mama." As parents become excited when a baby seems to be saying "dada" or "mama," the child learns that those sounds are apparently more important than the other sounds. This is how language begins.

Unfortunately, many children with severe language disorders, including those with early signs of autism, don't babble very much. And even if they do babble, they don't seem to care as much about adult attention as typically developing kids. Children with delays also don't tend to imitate actions, which is the way children learn to play. They don't verbally imitate or echo sounds or words as much either, which is how language is typically learned.

Children with delays who don't babble much or spontaneously make sounds and say words throughout the day may also have poor articulation, which means they have difficulty pronouncing words. This can make the little language they do have difficult to understand.

You might say that your child doesn't talk or communicate with you at all or is nonverbal. But everyone, including a newborn baby, is verbal. Babbling, using gestures, crying, and engaging in problem behaviors like tantrums are technically all forms of communication. The goal is to teach your child to be *vocal* and *verbal* so that he can talk and communicate with you and others more effectively.

Remember that language skills are both expressive and receptive. Expressive language or speech is made up of four elementary "verbal operants," which include *mands* or requests, *tacts* or labels, *echoics* or repeating what someone says, and *intraverbals* or the ability to answer questions. In this chapter, you'll learn the powerful combination of mands, tacts, and echoics. Since intra-verbal language doesn't emerge for typically developing children until about 18 months, we'll cover that operant in Chapter 9.

In addition to encouraging verbal behavior or expressive skills, I will also teach you in this chapter how to increase your child's ability to follow directions, imitate, and perform matching tasks, which are all very important to early and advanced language development.

But again, don't skip ahead even if your child is already following some directions and answering basic questions. Here's why: It's quite common for kids with autism or language delays to have scattered skills, so even if your child is talking, he may be missing some of the basic learning building blocks that you'll read about here. These communication and learning skills need to be strengthened so that your child can "learn to learn."

Let's talk about how to quickly assess your child's verbal and nonverbal behavior so that you can get going with increasing language starting today!

## ASSESSMENT AND PLAN: YOUR CHILD'S EARLY LANGUAGE SKILLS

You've already read the chapters on assessment and planning. The TAA assessment form we discussed in Chapter 4 helped you quickly assess your child's basic language capabilities. The two short videos, as well as the baseline language sample mentioned in that chapter, are also important assessment tools.

To look more closely at expressive language, the baseline language sample is used as our main tool during the assessment phase. This is where you'll keep more detailed language data by writing down the sounds, words, or phrases your child says in a 15-minute period, a 30-minute period, or a 60-minute period. Set a timer, and write down only what you hear during that time. Your sheet might include sounds like "da da da," words like "dog," or phrases like "give me that car."

As you can see from Elena's story, taking language samples at the beginning and then five weeks later was key! Through 60-minute time samples, Michelle was able to show that her daughter's language abilities went from 2 words to more than 180 words and phrases. This gave Michelle clear evidence that the time she spent at home teaching her daughter was successful, and they were heading in the right direction. These timed language samples also correlated nicely with Elena's pre- and post-standardized speech and language assessments.

In addition to the baseline language sample, if your child has any words, you might also want to create a list of sounds, word approximations, and/or words you hear your child say on a daily basis or at least words you heard once in the past week or two. Many children have what I call "pop out" words, which are words you hear at random times. While it's a good idea to keep track of "pop out" words and look for ways to increase the odds of hearing those words, resist the urge to write down words you heard three months ago. They will no longer be relevant.

From this list of sounds, words, and phrases, you'll be able to gather more clues. I was surprised to find out, for example, that my client Chino could say "Cheeto" when he wanted his favorite snack and could say "no," but he couldn't say "Chino" clearly until we taught him that skill. Learning the words your child can and can't say clearly will help you in many ways. If you learn that your child can say "star" while you sing "Twinkle, Twinkle, Little Star," you can then gather pictures of stars for teaching programs.

By writing down sounds and words your child is using even sporadically, you'll see whether he's using only vowels or if he's putting certain consonants and vowels together to make words. It's helpful to keep a spreadsheet so that you can keep sounds and words in alphabetical order as you add them.

Once your child starts to say more words, his articulation might not be great in all cases. So it's useful to keep two lists: (1) with words that he says clearly, and (2) with words that are approximations or sounds that aren't clear yet. A word approximation on list 2 might be "app-a," which he uses for "apple." If you prefer, you can keep both word lists on the refrigerator so that you can add to them easily as you hear new words and sounds during the day. This will also allow you to move list 2 words to list 1 once your child is able to clearly articulate them.

Let's say your child says 10 to 20 words either occasionally or on a regular basis. Pay attention to how he uses these words. Is he manding for the items? Is he labeling pictures? Is he echoing you by saying them?

You'll also need to assess your child's receptive abilities. If you completed the Turn Autism Around assessment form, you will already have assessed his ability to follow directions, such as touching body parts, clapping, or standing up without you demonstrating the action, as well as his baseline imitation and matching skills.

Since feeding, drinking issues, and even pacifier use can have a big impact on talking, be sure the assessment form is filled out to consider those areas, too. It's imperative that you complete the full assessment and planning forms and gather your materials before you proceed.

Now, let's move on to interventions to improve language!

## INTERVENTIONS: THE POWER OF LEARNING TIME AT THE TABLE

Toddlers and preschool children with significant delays need lots of learning opportunities in order to give them the best chance of catching up. I've found that the quicker you can get your child sitting at a table to learn, the better he will do.

Remember that you'll also need to sanitize the room or area where you will be having table time, removing your child's free access to toys or other potential items of interest in the room. This way, he will be more likely to want to stay with you and find the table and materials fun. And you'll need to gather the materials from the checklist in Chapter 5 before you can begin to implement the strategies in this chapter.

It's important to keep the learning materials in a bin or a locked closet or cabinet to be used for table time only. Also, for toys and materials that have parts such as Mr. Potato Head or inset puzzles, keep each set of parts in labeled clear bags or containers. Do not allow your child free access to these toys/materials when you're not with him at the table. If you do, the materials could easily become toys used for stimming, which means toys that he plays with repeatedly for self-stimulation.

## Pairing and Reinforcement

We already discussed pairing, but since it's such an important concept, I want to cover it more here and specifically tell you how to pair the learning area with good things. *Pairing* refers to using things the child likes (including bubbles, snacks, attention, etc.) and delivering these items without any demands being placed on your child. This will make you, the learning environment, the table, and the materials positive and fun. If your child is running to the table, smiles when he sees the reinforcing items, and is eager to sit and learn from you, you're on the right track. Pairing is not a one-time thing, though, so if your child resists sitting or doesn't like the items or activities, focus on re-pairing the table to make sure he *wants* to be there with you.

There are two main types of reinforcement: reinforcing items and praise. Reinforcing items may include a few edible items, a drink, an electronic device such as a tablet, and/or other items your child loves. Any object that your child likes can be used as a positive reinforcer.

Sometimes, however, children are so obsessed with an item or a tablet that it's best not to use it during learning time. You don't want your child to not like table time, so pick reinforcers that he likes or loves but is not obsessed with, especially in the beginning.

If your child tries to leave the table or the learning area, it probably means you don't have his strongest reinforcers at the table with you. If the room isn't sanitized, and you don't have his favorite things at the table, you're fighting an uphill battle to get him to sit, attend to the materials, and love learning with you.

So before you get out the bin of materials or try to have your child sit with you, the table needs to be well paired with reinforcement. Initially, start out with very short bursts of three to five minutes with you and your child at the table to pair the reinforcing items you've gathered.

Don't ever force your child to sit, and don't block him with your legs or hold him in the chair—*ever*. He should be free to leave the table, which is one of the reasons I don't recommend strapping kids in high chairs or booster seats for learning time unless they're unsafe at a child-size table or alternate seating has been specifically recommended by a professional.

If you still struggle to get him to stay at the table or learning area, be careful how you react. I don't recommend saying, "You have to come back here and sit down." Instead, become a detective. Watch where he goes and what he gravitates toward. Is he picking up a figurine that was left out in the room? Did he find a piece of string on the floor? Did he decide to sit in a rocking chair in the room? If so, try bringing those items to the table as reinforcers, or sanitize the room more thoroughly.

If your child leaves the table, let him go, but here's something important to remember: the learning materials and reinforcers need to stay *at the table* until he returns. If he's allowed to take the reinforcing items or the materials away from the table, the learning area is suddenly not as special. If your room is well sanitized, it shouldn't take your child long to figure out that he wants to be at the table engaging with you.

I'm also not a big fan of the "Let's work for a break" approach, because then your child is working to get away from you. I also don't like to say, "Three more, and then you get a break." I want the child to *run* to the table, the materials, the reinforcers, and *you*.

This might be a good time to repeat that I don't recommend you use the word "work" at all. Instead, call it "learning time," "table time," or "mommy fun time!"

For your first short table time sessions, your child should not be expected to do any "work" or even use any of the materials. He should get the reinforcers for "free" just for sitting at the table with you. If your child refuses to sit initially, deliver reinforcement as he stands next to the table. But don't expand teaching time past three minutes until your child willingly sits.

As you slowly increase the length of your table time teaching sessions up to 15 minutes, split your time between table time and other fun activities away from the table. You might do 10 or 15 minutes of table time followed by going outside or in the playroom.

But go with him during breaks from the table, which will include natural environment teaching as much as you can. It shouldn't be a break to get away from you. Try to make break time as engaging as possible, and give yourself a break if you need one. As you gain confidence during table time, you'll also learn how to use times throughout the day to work on things like manding, imitation, play skills, and generalization of skills while your child is at home, at school, and even in the community.

## Using Reinforcing Items to Get Your Child to Ask for What He Wants

The center of all of your teaching programs at the table and everything you do with your child should be *manding* or requesting. This is because when he's motivated and wants something, you have the best chance of teaching him new skills. When he's able to communicate what he wants and tell you and others, it will make a huge difference in both your lives.

As we discussed in Chapter 6, problem behaviors are almost always a result of a child's inability to mand, whether verbally or nonverbally. Problem behaviors are, in their own way, a type of mand, just as crying is a newborn baby's way of manding.

A child has to be motivated to mand for something, however. In Chapter 5, you learned about the One Word x3 Strategy, pairing words up to three times with the item your child wants. But he must *want* the item before he can learn to ask for it. Therefore, in the beginning, the items that you'll use to pair the table and eventually teach your child to ask for should be strong reinforcers that he's motivated to get. These reinforcing items might be a ball, juice, cookies, a tablet, or a short clip of a video.

Be careful to control the reinforcement while at the table, and don't allow your child to grab items or access them without your help. I've found that using clear containers that are difficult to open instead of bowls to hold edible reinforcements are best. Give your child the items one at a time as you pair the word with the item. For electronics, I recommend 10- to 30-second clips of a movie or a short video using a tablet after pairing the word "movie" or "video." If your child can't yet ask for things by talking or signing, just continue to pair the word up to three times before delivery.

At the table, you can teach manding by breaking up or dividing an item into pieces. Assuming your child likes or loves apples, you could cut an apple into 10 pieces so that he has 10 opportunities at the table to say "apple." Hold the piece of apple to your chin and say "apple, apple, apple" slowly and in an animated way. Then give him the piece of apple. After you've tried this a couple of times, wait two to three seconds before providing the piece of apple in order to give him the chance to mand for it.

You can also bring the piece of apple closer to him as you say "apple, apple, apple" and then pull it away slightly to see if he will mand for it. If he reaches for the apple without saying "apple," give him the piece of apple. If he says "ah" or "ap," that's certainly progress, so give him the piece of apple right after he says any word approximation for it.

If your child likes cookies, grapes, pepperoni, or chips, break or cut them into several pieces. This gives you more opportunities for him to mand. Hold one piece of a cookie up to your chin, and say "cookie, cookie, cookie." If he loses interest in cookies, try one of the other reinforcing items.

Don't ever say, "If you want a cookie, you have to say 'cookie.'" Even if your child can talk and you heard him say "cookie" yesterday, requiring spoken words isn't a good idea since there's no way you can "make" a child (or anyone else, for that matter) say anything. Instead, keep your interactions with your child positive, and don't get into a power struggle. Just say the word up to three times, and deliver it (as long as your child is not exhibiting any problem behaviors).

Once your child has learned to mand for items that are in sight, place those items slightly farther away so that he will hopefully ask for them. After he has manded several times for a particular item that's slightly farther away and is still motivated to have it, try placing it under the table or hiding it behind something on the table. He may need you to show him where it is before he will mand for it, though. If that doesn't work, you can bring it back into sight and try placing it out of sight again later.

Continue to teach manding throughout the day whenever you see an opportunity, such as at the dinner table or when you're outside playing. Bubbles are often highly reinforcing for young children, so if your child enjoys bubbles, he might mand for the bottle of liquid or for you to blow the bubbles.

You may be tempted to try to teach your child to say "more" or "please" when learning to mand, but I discourage this with young children who have language delays. Instead, concentrate on teaching him the words for concrete objects he desires. If your child learns "more" or "please" and only says one of those words, you'll have no idea what he's asking for, especially if the item is out of sight. If he learns "cookie," however, you'll know exactly what he wants.

Some children will begin to mand quickly, while others will take longer. Don't get discouraged; just keep working with your child by giving him many opportunities throughout the day to mand for his favorite things. You do this by making sure he's motivated to request it because it's out of reach.

## Sign Language

If you are trying to teach your child to mand but are getting few or no sounds or word approximations, consider teaching him sign language. Teaching kids to use signs to request items can often be a springboard to vocal language, and it can also improve imitation skills, prevent or reduce problem behaviors, and increase a child's toleration of gentle physical prompts. Many professionals believe that children need to imitate before they can learn sign language, but I've found that teaching children to sign is one of the best ways to teach them to imitate. Some people also worry that sign language prevents children with delays from speaking, but in my experience, when signing is accompanied by spoken words, it almost always improves vocalizations.

To get started with signs, it's best to focus on teaching three to five at a time. When your child wants a "ball," you can first teach him to mand for it using sign language by holding up the ball, making the sign yourself, helping your child make the sign, and then delivering the ball to him. During each step, say "ball" while you and your child make the sign for ball so that your child hears "ball" three or four times before it's delivered.

If you physically prompt a child's hand to make the sign for "chip" and give him the reinforcement of a chip right away, you have paired your teaching and physical prompts with reinforcement, which will help your child learn all sorts of skills.

There are also speech devices and apps to help nonverbal children communicate. While I encourage the early use of sign language, I'm not as big a fan of using these speech devices with very young children, at least not in the beginning. However, if your child is already using a tablet app or another augmentative system for communicating and having some success, I would continue with that system. I would also start using the Turn Autism Around approach to see if the combination might help boost vocal language and increase other communication skills, while reducing problem behaviors.

## Teaching Talking (and Following Directions) at the Table: Using a Shoebox, Flashcards, and Pictures

Now that you have your child coming to the table to accept small bites of food, sips of a favorite drink, bubbles, and short clips of a favorite movie, it might be time to introduce some of the other materials you have gathered. I say "might be time" because if your child is still refusing to sit or whining when he sees the table, it's probably not paired up enough to introduce additional materials, which he could view as "work." But if your child is willingly coming and sitting with you for three to five minutes at the table and getting reinforcement with no demands, you both are probably ready for more materials.

As you introduce these new items, you'll need to continue to have your child's reinforcing items (the ones you already gathered for manding) always at the table. You'll deliver the reinforcement frequently while you pair up the new materials.

Best of all, once you learn how to use the materials, table time in general will actually become a powerful reinforcer on its own. This means you'll require fewer external reinforcers over time.

Most children, especially those who have language delays, enjoy visual tasks with a cause and an effect. This is why I developed the shoebox program. Cut a large slit into the lid of a shoebox. With the shoebox on the table, hold a flashcard or photo up to your chin or by your face, and say the name of the pictured object up to three times slowly in an animated tone, such as "cat, cat, cat." Focus on the vowels, and elongate them slightly when you speak.

Each time you say the word, move the picture closer to your child. In the beginning, you might need to gently take your child's hand and help him place the card in the slit in the box. He will soon learn to put the card in the box by himself, and believe it or not, the simple act of putting the card in the box often becomes reinforcing.

If your child says the word, this word is actually part mand (because he wants the item or picture to put it in the box), part tact (because he can see the item or picture), and part echoic (because he's verbally imitating you). This is called *multiple control*, which means we combine two or more operants (mands, tacts, and/or echoics) to improve learning. The TAA approach uses *multiple control* procedures in each activity.

Remember, however, that while you might turn your child's chair so that he's facing you, don't put his body into a position to try to force eye contact. If your child isn't yet talking, I would prefer he starts looking at your mouth and your whole face rather than your eyes so that he sees how words are formed. For this reason, I recommend you continue holding items and pictures next to your mouth and chin, which should encourage your child to look at your face. Over time, this procedure should naturally improve joint attention, too.

## Using Mr. Potato Head

Mr. Potato Head is also recommended for your learning sessions and is one of the best toys for teaching body parts. Hold up one part at a time next to your mouth. As you hold up the nose, say "nose, nose, nose" slowly as you bring the nose to your child's hand. In the beginning, you may need to guide his hand to put the nose in the right place on Mr. Potato Head's face.

After your child likes the Mr. Potato Head activity, you can try touching your own nose, then physically prompting your child very gently to touch his own nose. If he resists your physical prompts, the skill might be too hard, or you might be prompting too much. But if he starts to touch his own nose after seeing you touch yours, his imitation skills are also building, which is *huge*!

## Using Toys and Books

You can use the cause-and-effect toys you've gathered to work on talking, too. For a hammer and ball toy, you could say "ball" as you hand your child each of the four balls to put in the holes and then say "hammer" as you hand him the hammer so that he can hit each ball. If your child says "ball" or "hammer," these words are part mand, part tact, and part echoic, just like the shoebox activity. Be careful about labeling colors, though, as trying to teach colors too soon is a common mistake that we'll discuss in the next chapter.

You can also use first word books and other simple books you have gathered to encourage both receptive and expressive language at the table. In the beginning, just label one picture per page. Eventually, ask your child to touch certain pictures to improve his ability to comprehend and follow directions.

## Teaching Matching: Using Inset Puzzles, Flashcards, and Pictures

To teach matching, you'll need to start with the simple inset puzzles you have gathered. Hold up one puzzle piece at a time, and label the word up to three times. Then help your child match the puzzle piece with the empty space where it belongs. For an animal puzzle, hold up the pig next to your mouth, and say "pig, pig, pig" slowly, as you bring the pig closer to your child each time until you hand it to him and help him put the piece in the correct spot (or watch him do it by himself). If your child says "pig" after you say it one time, make sure to give him the puzzle piece immediately!

You can also use the two identical sets of first word flashcards that you purchased or the pictures of reinforcing items and people so that your child can learn to match the pictures. In the beginning, keep the number of pictures on the table to two or three, and don't use pictures of only animals or only vehicles, which could be confusing. For example, lay out pictures of a car, mommy, and a bed. Then hold up the matching picture for car and say "car."

For matching tasks, many professionals recommend you say "match" or "match car," but I recommend you only say "match" when you're assessing matching skills. To teach matching, I suggest using the item name only. This way you'll work on more than just matching during these activities. You will pair up the child's desire to match so that he'll want to take the picture from you and match it. Because he wants to match the picture, even though it's a matching program, you'll also be working on your child's ability to mand for the picture of the car, as well as his tacting and echoic skills.

If your child echoes a word during a matching activity, I want that word to be the item name (in this case "car") and not the word "match" or the phrase "match car." If he struggles to make the match, you can say, "Car goes here," and help him place the card on top of its matching card until he can do it himself.

Before you begin matching or any of the early learner programs, decide what label you'll give to yourself and other people, pictures, and items. If your child can say "Ma" and "Mama" but can't say "Mommy" yet, then I'd pair "Mama" three times to start. Once your child learns to talk and echo, you can transition to "Mommy" or "Mom." For matching, hold up the picture and say "Mama" three times, moving the photo from next to your chin toward your child, and then place it in your child's hands. He doesn't have to say "Mama" to get the picture to match, but if he does, give him lots of extra praise and a reinforcement.

## Teaching Imitation Skills: Using Identical Objects

As I said earlier, typically developing children learn language, play, and social skills through imitation. Lack of imitation is a red flag for autism and a core deficit for many children who have speech delays. Imitation is usually easier for children than following directions. A child will be able to touch his head, for example, with the visual prompt of you touching your head before he can respond to the simple verbal command, "Touch your head."

To teach imitation skills at the table, I recommend starting with the identical objects you've gathered. You might have, for example, two identical cars, forks, spoons, and cups—a set for each of you. As you place your spoon into your cup, say, "Do this." Then if your child is unable to do it on his own, gently take his hands and help him put his spoon into his cup. You could then say, "Do this," as you stir the spoon in the cup. You might then have two small dolls on the table to feed with the spoons. In this way, your child will learn that a spoon can do more than one thing. He will also learn that imitation of skills leads to reinforcement, which will increase the behavior you want.

You can also teach imitation with two identical toy cars. Say, "Do this," and move the car back and forth. Then guide his hand to imitate you with his car. Eventually, he should begin to imitate you without prompting.

After your child has begun to imitate actions with objects, try getting him to imitate your body movements, such as clapping, putting your hands up, or patting the table. First, demonstrate clapping in front of him or with both of you standing in front of a full-length mirror, and provide some level of prompting or help if needed. Then provide an immediate reinforcement.

## GETTING YOUR CHILD TO RESPOND TO HIS NAME

One of the red flags for autism is that a child doesn't respond to his name, but this is something you can teach him.

First of all, I recommend that all adults around your child avoid overusing your child's name, as you don't want him to tune it out. So stop using his name frequently, especially when you say "no" or "stop." You can continue to use your child's name during a fun activity, such as when you're pushing him on the swing or when delivering praise or another reinforcement.

To help him learn to respond to his name, gather several of his favorite reinforcers, and while he's involved in some activity, call his name from right behind him. Then immediately (and gently) touch his shoulder and hand him a reinforcement.

He will begin to learn that he gets something good when he hears his name. You can do this periodically throughout the day—gradually stand farther away as you call his name. Then give him a couple of seconds before you approach, touch his shoulder, and offer the reinforcement.

## NEVER GIVE UP

Teaching language and other skills to your child can be a slow process. Some children, like Elena, learn very quickly, while others will take longer. Sometimes, you'll struggle with teaching your child, only to have the floodgates open. Whatever you do, *never give up*.

In the next chapter, you'll learn about more advanced communication skills and the common mistakes both parents and professionals make, along with what to do instead.

# CHAPTER 9

# Talking but Not Conversational: Strategies to Expand Language

Three-year-old Drew is the younger brother of my former client Sam, who got lost while he and his parents were visiting the Statue of Liberty. Since Drew's risk of autism was high as the sibling of a child with autism, his parents watched his development carefully and felt that he was on track for his first two and a half years. But as soon as Drew turned three, which coincided with a three-month break in his daycare placement, his physician mom began to panic as his language skills appeared to regress.

She was desperate for me to assess Drew and tell her if I thought he had autism. She needed to know what to do. Should she get him on a waiting list to be evaluated by a speech pathologist? Should she seek an evaluation by a developmental pediatrician? Was she only worrying because he turned three that week? Were her expectations too high? Was his language regressing because he wasn't exposed to typically developing peers? Or were they too busy and failing to provide him with enough engagement?

When I arrived at Drew's house, I was happy to see that he had good eye contact and said, "Hi, Miss Mary," when prompted by his mother. While his mom and I chatted about the Turn Autism

Around assessment form she completed that day, Drew climbed up to a keyboard and threw the music books on the floor. He looked back and forth at me and his mom, clearly trying to get our attention. Even though throwing things is technically problem behavior, in this case, I was almost relieved to see him seeking our attention in a somewhat typical way.

I started pulling things from my bag to start the Screening Tool for Autism in Toddlers (STAT), which I talked about in the first chapter. I pulled out a ball and a car for the first test activity, and Drew chose the "yellow racing car," which wasn't surprising because his mom told me he was "obsessed" with cars and trucks. He sat with his mom, and we rolled the car back and forth five times, which led to Drew easily passing the first STAT subtest.

The trouble started when I wanted to put the car away and pulled out the doll materials next. Drew cried, grabbed at the car (which I wouldn't give him), and proceeded to throw himself on the floor as he cried for a few minutes.

Transitioning from one activity to another was difficult for Drew, even when it didn't involve cars. While he passed almost all the subtests and used several full sentences when he was calm, such as "I want to do it myself" and "Make it go up to the roof" when I flew a spinning toy near the ceiling, he communicated a lot with problem behaviors. And when he threw a tantrum, he used single words like "mine" and "car" instead of talking in sentences.

Drew's parents were surprised by his tantrums, however. They said his behavior almost never escalated to flopping on the floor. I explained that they were inadvertently reinforcing their son's problem behaviors by giving Drew items when he was crying and talking to him while he displayed more minor problem behaviors. I knew this was the case because while Drew was crying and flopping in front of us, both of his parents were using bribery tactics instead of reinforcement procedures like we discussed earlier. They said things like, "That's Miss Mary's yellow car. We'll buy you a yellow car at the store tomorrow." Drew's escalation of problem behaviors also made it clear that they were giving him things when he was crying to "turn off" the crying. When I didn't give him the car when he cried, his behaviors got worse.

They are both established professionals and caring parents, and I had worked with them for a few years in the past to help Drew's older brother, whose needs and behaviors looked very different. They were embarrassed when I pointed out that they were unknowingly reinforcing Drew's tantrums, which was also affecting his language.

Even though Drew passed the STAT test for toddlers and most likely will not be diagnosed with autism, I'll tell you later in this chapter what I recommended for Drew's worried parents.

Landon's language comprehension was poor, but he could script lines from movies. His mother Nicole was concerned that he didn't use functional language to request things he wanted, and the gap between his development and that of his typically developing peers seemed to grow bigger every day. He also exhibited problem behaviors when his mom tried to teach him anything. He would throw himself out of his chair rather than sit and attend to learning.

Landon was three and a half years old and hadn't yet been diagnosed with autism, as he had been on a waiting list for more than nine months to be evaluated by a developmental pediatrician. Nicole was very worried by the time she found my Turn Autism Around program online.

Drew and Landon had a lot in common. They were both three years old and talking, but not conversational when their moms completed the TAA assessment and planning forms. They both exhibited a lot of problem behaviors, which they were using instead of advanced language to communicate. Neither of the boys had a diagnosis when their parents started implementing the Turn Autism Around strategies, although Landon did go on to receive an autism diagnosis before he turned four.

If, like Drew and Landon or even like two-year-old Elena from the previous chapter, your child is talking with single words or short phrases but not yet conversational, your work is far from done. Most typical children talk in full sentences by the time they're three, they start to tell simple stories, and are fully conversational by the age of four. But with children who have language delays, we can't just cross our fingers and hope they become conversational without our help.

Sure, some kids will catch up on their own, but many children with autism or language delays need systematic instruction to catch up their basic language. This is the only way some kids will become more verbal and conversational.

Many parents and professionals (including me in the past) try to teach language that's too difficult, however, which inadvertently contributes to the development of problem behaviors like Drew's and/or weird language that isn't functional, which we saw with Landon's scripting.

If your child is speaking in short phrases, you may be eager to jump ahead and try to get him to talk in full sentences. You may want to get him naming colors and adding prepositions and pronouns in his vocabulary. But resist the urge to pass by the prerequisites. The fact that your child is talking is a great sign, but it's important to build language in the right order. Like building a house that needs a solid foundation, you can't build advanced language on an unstable base.

Nevertheless, teaching kids who are talking but not yet conversational is very tricky, and there's a limit to what I can include in a book like this. Because of the complexity, this chapter will simply give you some guidelines to build advanced language and get you started.

If your child has some language skills, I highly recommend that you learn more (check out TurnAutismAround.com). I also suggest that you try to get at least one professional to help you, preferably someone who has been trained in the Turn Autism Around approach, if at all possible.

## WHAT IS CONVERSATION?

As functioning adults, we take conversation for granted. We learned it naturally, and we don't think about its complexities unless and until we try to learn a foreign language or try to teach a child with language delays.

Let's evaluate the anatomy of a casual conversation. Pretend that the two of us are sitting next to each other at a conference, and I strike up a conversation with you. I might not ask you directly about yourself, but I might say something like, "It's a beautiful day" or "This room is cold." In essence, I'm trying to get your attention (manding), as well as tacting (labeling) the environment.

If you're interested in having a conversation with me, you'll also make a comment or ask me a question such as, "Where are you from?"

I answer, "Pennsylvania. What about you?"

You answer, "California."

A conversation is really just a series of advanced mands for attention and information followed by advanced intraverbals. We use advanced intraverbal language to answer questions, and this also requires advanced comprehension.

When you're trying to learn a foreign language, intraverbal language is the most difficult verbal operant to learn. You have to understand what someone else is asking you in complete sentences. Then you have to know the language well enough to answer them correctly. So in the beginning, you need your instructor to take it slow until you know enough words and grammar rules to understand complex questions and have the ability to answer in full sentences.

For our children with language delays, we also have to be mindful of working on the right skills in the correct order based on each child's strengths and needs.

## ASSESSMENTS: FINDING YOUR STARTING POINT

No matter how high functioning your child seems to be or what evaluations have already been done, the TAA assessment and planning forms from Chapters 4 and 5 are important to give you a quick look at your whole child to ensure you're focusing on the right goals.

For children who are starting with more intermediate or advanced language skills or for children who have progressed to this level using early learner programs, additional assessments may be needed to adequately determine their language skills. Only then can you create a plan and know what goals to select.

You saw in the last chapter how helpful it was for Elena's mom to receive standardized speech evaluations right before and after implementing the Turn Autism Around approach. Standardized speech evaluations are even more critical for children like Drew, whose language seems pretty typical, or for those like Landon who might have scattered skills.

It's also ideal to complete (or have a professional complete) the full VB-MAPP published by Dr. Mark Sundberg. The VB-MAPP includes three parts: milestones, barriers, and transition assessment. It can take hours to complete, as well as some skills to do it, and the higher your child's language skills, the more time and expertise you or the professional will need to complete it correctly.

The VB-MAPP assessment is comprehensive and was created based on milestones of typically developing children from birth to 4 years of age. Level 1 consists of the early learner skills of a typical 0- to 18-month-old child, Level 2 includes the intermediate learner skills of 18- to 30-month-olds, and Level 3 includes the preschool skills of 30- to 48-month-olds.

Information about purchasing the electronic or paper version of the VB-MAPP assessment can be found at TurnAutismAround .com. I recommend the electronic version, which will automatically generate a report for you, as well as provide you with recommended goals. You can update it and get a score in each area at the same time as you update the TAA assessment (every few months or at least annually). This way, you can easily see your child's progress.

## PLANNING: THE IMPORTANCE OF PICKING THE RIGHT GOALS

Before you picked up this book, you probably thought all assessments, planning, and goals for your child were the job of professionals. But now that you know you have an important role in helping your child, you're more aware of the dangers of working on the wrong goals or trying to teach your child skills that are too hard.

I told you a little bit about Lucas's first speech therapy sessions, but now that you know more about verbal behavior and the Turn Autism Around approach, I'll tell you more about those early sessions. This will illustrate the importance of making sure your plan is based on your child's individualized assessments, as well as the goals you and any professionals select.

Lucas started weekly speech sessions when he was two, shortly after he began attending the toddler preschool class. This was way before I knew anything about autism or verbal behavior and almost a year before Lucas's autism diagnosis when I was hoping and praying it was just a speech delay. My husband and I were fairly optimistic (me more so than him) that the combination of preschool and weekly speech sessions would help Lucas catch up.

I always brought my son to his speech sessions, and most of the time, I was able to be in the room watching the speech and language pathologist (SLP) work with him during the 30-minute sessions. If I had to bring my younger son, Spencer, along, I'd watch the sessions from a two-way glass mirror in the next room.

The SLP would always start the session with a fun activity like bubbles or use another cause-and-effect type of toy. Back then, Lucas had "pop out" words, but I had no idea how to teach him to say those words or any other words on demand. So I watched his speech sessions closely to learn from an expert how to get Lucas to talk. During the fun activities, the SLP could usually get Lucas to say some words like "bubble" and "blow."

Years later when I became a BCBA, I realized that these types of activities were pairing and manding sessions. I also learned that when Lucas said "bubble," it was *multiple controlled* or occurred for multiple reasons.

I'm positive neither the SLP nor I knew the term *multiple control* back then. But Lucas saying the word "bubble" during the fun activity was part mand (because he wanted her to open the container and blow toward the wand), part tact (because the bubbles were in sight), and part echoic (since the SLP said the word right before she opened or blew the bubbles).

Lucas loved the first part of his speech sessions and did well. The problems began when the fun activity ended abruptly, and they moved on to working on his more difficult abstract language goals.

One activity related to the quantity language goal and involved the SLP introducing a few small piles of objects. She then attempted to have Lucas give her "one," "some," or "all" of the items. Another difficult goal was for Lucas to shake his head or say "yes" and "no" appropriately. The SLP held up various pictures one at a time and asked Lucas questions like, "Is this an apple?" which required a "yes" or "no" response. The SLP also worked on pronouns like "my turn" and "your turn" while playing simple games, but Lucas didn't understand any game rules, let alone how to use pronouns. She also tried to teach Lucas prepositions by asking him to put the doll "next to" or "in" the bed.

Fortunately, even though the majority of goals and activities during the sessions were too difficult for Lucas, he didn't have any problem behaviors like crying or whining. I practically begged the SLP for "homework"—books I could read or videos I could watch to help Lucas in between sessions—but she couldn't point me toward any resources. We didn't know it at the time, but we were making the number one mistake I still see both parents and professionals make: trying to teach Lucas skills that were far too difficult.

He didn't fuss when she put the bubbles away and transitioned to these difficult concepts. He was simply confused and unable to respond. The SLP sessions should have included *only* fun activities like the bubble-blowing in which Lucas's words were part mand, part tact, and part echoic. Until he was echoing us throughout the day, we shouldn't have even attempted to work on more advanced and abstract goals such as yes/no tacts, pronouns, or prepositions.

We should have focused on the *one thing that could have made all the difference.* I'm confident this one thing—gaining echoic control—would have opened up the language floodgates.

## THE POWER OF DEVELOPING ECHOIC CONTROL

When most ABA professionals talk about *echoic control*, they mean sitting across from a child at a table and saying words or phrases that the child echoes. So a therapist says, "Say ball," and the child says "ball" without a ball or a picture of a ball present.

But the Turn Autism Around approach to gaining echoic control involves using the early learner materials and "multiple control" strategies to combine mands, tacts, and echoics. Using the flashcards and the shoebox, we hold up pictures of reinforcing items or people one at a time and say each word up to three times. Eventually, the table time sessions using the early learner materials from the checklist and "multiple control" procedures usually result in some echoing. This should then start spilling over until your child echoes you throughout the day with items in and out of sight. This is the best way I've found to establish echoic control.

If there is one thing I've learned over the years about teaching language, it's that without imitation (especially verbal imitation or echoic skills), it's hard to teach children any new skills.

As we've discussed, imitation is the way typically developing babies and toddlers learn language. They babble, and because Mom gets super excited to hear "mama" or "baba" for bottle, the baby soon realizes certain sounds or words lead to getting things and getting adults to make silly faces and smile. By 18 months, kids usually echo or repeat what adults and other kids say.

So if your child doesn't echo you yet (whether he's completely silent or has "pop out" words), use all the materials and techniques in the previous chapter to try to get him to say more words every day. In most cases, after days, weeks, or months of short daily sessions, parents do get their children to echo them. Once a child starts to echo, the pace of progress usually quickens, and the language floodgates often open.

## GET LANGUAGE ON THE RIGHT TRACK BY FIXING ERRORS

If your child is scripting from movies like Landon, or using hundreds of one- and two-word utterances like Elena, they most likely already have echoic control. But you might have different problems. Your child's language may be full of errors like pronoun reversals where he says, "You want a cookie," or "Pick you up," instead of "I want a cookie," and "Pick me up." He may be confused like Lucas was in his speech sessions and say "yes" when he means "no." Your child may be speaking in sentences at times like Drew, but using tantrums to communicate at other times. Or he may be able to recite the whole alphabet without the ability to tact Mom versus Dad or answer simple questions.

If your child's language isn't progressing and/or his language sounds "weird," it's probably because he doesn't understand language fully and hasn't learned basic and abstract language skills in the correct order. He may also have a lot of scattered skills, making it difficult for you and professionals to decipher how high functioning he really is and what strategies might help get his language unstuck.

It will probably take some work on your part, as well as your child's team, to undo some of the scripting and language errors that are holding your child back from making meaningful progress. Be sure to complete the TAA assessment and plan, and ensure that any goals for your child are based on his unique strengths and needs. It might also be a good idea to have a professional complete the VB-MAPP assessment; but in the meantime, the TAA forms will help you. It's likely that once you review your assessment, plan, and current goals, you'll need to partner with any professionals currently working with your child to revise all goals that are too hard. It may feel like you're taking a step backward, but trust me—goals and programs that are too hard aren't good for you or your child.

That said, the fact that your child's language is filled with errors or not improving is no one's fault, including yours. You and every person who has ever worked with your child wants what is best for him. For years, I made all the mistakes I'm going to cover in the next section, and I didn't know how to teach conversational skills for a full decade after falling into the autism world.

Unlike the previous or upcoming chapters, though, I won't provide as much step-by-step guidance in this chapter. This is because programming for intermediate learners who are talking but not yet conversational is so complicated. The goals and programs I would recommend for Elena, Drew, and Landon would all be very different and specific to their individual assessments.

Nevertheless, there are general recommendations and a few steps that will hold true for all intermediate or advanced language learners. But before I talk about those, let's review some of the most common mistakes I see when teaching language.

## Mistake 1: Focusing on the Length of Phrases and Sentences

Once we get the child talking, we have echoic control, and the child is saying some words, we need to expand language carefully. But instead, many parents push too hard, wanting desperately for their children to improve, and professionals select goals for four- or five-word-length sentences.

This desire to have your child communicate in full sentences often leads to the use of speech-generating devices and augmentative systems for young children who are nonverbal or minimally verbal. While I'm not opposed to these systems and devices for children who are not yet speaking, I caution you against focusing on expanding the length of utterance, which is the length of phrases or sentences, or setting goals for advancing higher language without a strong focus on improving vocal language.

When SLPs, BCBAs, teachers, and other professionals try to get kids to speak in complete sentences, they often teach what are called "carrier phrases." These are phrases such as "I want," "I need," "I see," and "That's a . . ." They encourage or even require children to add this carrier phrase in front of mands to form sentences like, "I want banana," or "I want bubble."

Throughout my years as a behavior analyst, I've seen carrier phrases backfire hundreds of times. If a child is not spontaneously manding frequently throughout the day, requiring him to request in a short sentence can lead him to become dependent upon prompts and can kill spontaneity. Here's an example of what can happen when carrier phrases are required: Timmy says "chip," but instead of being given a chip as a reinforcement, he's told, "Tell me like a big boy," or "Use your sentence to tell Mommy what you want." This often leads to a decrease of spontaneous mands and a dependency on adults prompting a child to say it differently with more words.

Adding carrier phrases also increases the number of syllables the child has to say, and this often causes articulation errors. "I want pretzel" might come out "I-wah pre-za," for example. As we discussed, it's important to pay attention to syllables when choosing any words or sentences you teach your child. You might think "refrigerator" would be easy to say because it's only one word, while "I want cracker" would be harder since it's three words. But "I want cracker" is just four syllables, while "refrigerator" is *five* syllables.

Children with few receptive language skills also have difficulty discriminating one carrier phrase from another, so they frequently get confused and use the wrong one. They might say, "I see juice," when they mean "I want juice." Or they might say, "I want cow," instead of "I see cow." They might also be confused about when to use a carrier phrase and when not to use one, leading to more functional errors that you have to work to correct.

Faith learned the carrier phrase "That's a . . ." at one point, which proved to be a problem. When we held up a picture of a cat or a ball and asked, "What is it?" she answered "That's a cat," and "That's a ball," instead of "cat" and "ball" as we'd taught her. Faith's ABA therapist didn't even notice that Faith had started to put "That's a . . ." in front of her tacts. When I asked the therapist who taught Faith to use that carrier phrase, she told me that Faith had recently started working with a new private speech therapist who'd probably taught it to her.

When I showed her a picture of herself and asked, "Who's this?" she answered, "That's a Faith." When I showed her a picture of a boy sleeping and asked, "What's he doing?" she answered, "That's a sleeping." You can see how these phrases can cause confusion and what we call *conditional discrimination errors*, which is when children have difficulty discriminating between similar things. In this case, Faith couldn't discriminate when to use "That's a . . ." and when not to use it, which resulted in errors.

For kids who speak in one- or two-syllable word utterances and who are echoic, here's my recommendation: Be careful with expanding into sentences. The goal should be teaching and encouraging a child to use one- or two-syllable words first before moving to three- and four-syllable words and two-word phrases, which might include actions (throw ball), plurals (Mommy's car), and adjectives (red bike). And as you expand language very carefully, make sure your child's articulation remains as clear as possible.

It's a natural assumption that the more words a child strings together, the more progress he's making. But if we teach children with autism to speak in a rote and rigid way, they won't develop flexible vocal language, and their progress toward becoming conversational will likely be sidetracked.

## Mistake 2: Not Knowing How to Deal with Scripting

*Delayed echolalia* or scripting is another issue that's common in children with autism who have some language but are not conversational. Scripting involves the repeating of words or phrases without understanding their meaning. It usually occurs because it's automatically reinforcing, but kids may also script to get attention or to get out of a difficult demand.

If a child scripts, it does show that he can speak, and if his words are understandable, it also shows that his articulation is pretty good. But scripting may make you think your child has more advanced language abilities than he does.

Lucas's delayed echolalia made me think his language was progressing and caused me to stay in denial longer. When Lucas was about 21 months old, we would take him to the park, and my husband, Charles, would point to the signs and say, "Please do not feed the ducks," adding "quack quack" at the end. Lucas loved going to the park and looking at the signs, but he never repeated any words since we didn't have echoic control and had no idea what that meant. After doing this a few times, however, Lucas started waking up in the middle of the night to say, "Please do not feed the ducks, quack, quack." I had no idea this was "delayed echolalia" or "scripting." We thought this was a sign of intelligence and didn't know it could be an early sign of autism.

When I asked the pediatrician how many words Lucas should be able to say, he said at least 25 words at 21 months old. I counted all the "pop out" words I'd heard in the prior few months and also included the 8 words from the park script (Please do not feed the ducks, quack, quack) to get up to 25 words. I used these nonfunctional words to justify or rationalize my stance that Lucas was fine and didn't need any evaluations or therapy.

Scripting is a sign that your child most likely needs a new assessment, a revised plan, and different goals.

## Mistake 3: Not Knowing How to Prevent or Correct Language Errors

As children begin to learn more language, they often confuse items that are similar. If you try to teach your child to distinguish between a pen and a pencil or between a chair, a sofa, and a stool, he may struggle.

One of the advanced skills is learning the features and functions of objects. Features would include the wheels, windshield, and doors of a car or the keyboard, screen, and mouse of a computer.

Functions involve learning what an airplane does or what you do with a cup. These are very complicated language skills, so be careful not to jump into these until your child has completed the necessary prerequisites on the VB-MAPP. Otherwise, you're likely to get errors.

As you teach your child the tact for "toothbrush," for example, you may also be adding information like, "Time to brush your teeth," "Your toothbrush has a red handle," or "Get the toothpaste." But then the next time you ask your child to identify a toothbrush, he might say, "Brush your teeth." I've seen that happen numerous times.

Just like the previous mistakes, don't feel bad if your child makes these errors. Before this chapter is finished, I'll give you some steps to follow, including the concept of "errorless teaching" to start helping your child's language improve.

## Mistake 4: Hyperfocusing on Colors and Other Pre-Academic Skills

I once assessed a boy who said "yellow chair" when asked, "What's this called?" as I pointed to the yellow chair. His parents were so proud of him because he had not only labeled the chair, but also its color. The problem is that it wasn't an appropriate answer to the question because I hadn't asked him the color of the chair. A typical child would probably just say "chair." You might not think this is a big deal, but it can cause issues as we expand to teach big versus little, the parts of a chair, and what we do with a chair.

In addition to avoiding abstract concepts such as pronouns, prepositions, and features, I also urge you not to rush to teach children to label colors, numbers, letters, or shapes. Typically developing kids usually start to identify colors and learn other pre-academic skills at 30 to 48 months. Because of this, it's a Level 3 VB-MAPP skill.

These pre-academic skills are more abstract than how to mand for and tact concrete objects and pictures. Pre-academics require higher conditional discrimination skills, which means your child may get confused between numbers six and nine or have difficulty tacting colors that are similar like orange versus red. Children who do not have delays pick up language naturally, including learning the names of colors without a lot of instruction, but this is often not the case for children with delays. So be patient, and try not to hyperfocus on teaching these skills if your child isn't ready for them.

## Mistake 5: Focusing Too Much on Talking While Neglecting Other Areas

When Lucas was diagnosed with an expressive and receptive language delay at age two and then with moderate-to-severe autism at three, I focused almost all my attention on teaching him to talk and expanding his expressive language skills. If Lucas talked more with different words or longer phrases, I thought he was doing better.

I made the mistake of focusing too much on measuring progress based on how much he was talking, and I often see this same mistake by both parents and professionals.

While expressive language is certainly important, older children and adults spend a lot of their days listening, learning, completing self-care tasks like showering and eating, and quietly entertaining themselves with leisure activities such as reading a book or exercising. So these nonverbal skills are also very important and should be a big part of your child's overall program.

Now that we've reviewed the five most common mistakes when trying to teach conversational skills to children, I'll give you three steps you can take to prevent and fix errors as you help your child's language progress.

## VIDEO MODELING

My former client Kurt was two years old when I started working with him more than a decade ago. Several times a day, he engaged in problem behaviors that were both aggressive and self-injurious. He didn't talk regularly, but he had a few pop out words.

I worked with him for about four months, and during a two-hour consultation, he would say about 10 words that were primarily tacts for body parts due to our work with Mr. Potato Head.

After months of weekly sessions, we still didn't have echoic control. We needed to increase his use of words, however, so I decided to try video modeling. I was taking a couple of weeks off for the holidays, so I made two short videos for Kurt. In one, I had his mom take a video of me touching my body parts as I said, "Eyes, nose, mouth, teeth, glasses," and ended that video with "hi" while waving. In the second short video, I sang, "Head, Shoulders, Knees, and Toes." I asked his mother to put them on his tablet, but then I forgot about them.

When I returned after the holidays and said hi to Kurt, he immediately said, "Hi. Eyes, nose, mouth, teeth, glasses. Hi!"

Obviously, he had watched the videos because he recited the body parts in the same order I recorded them. That day, instead of getting 10 words from him in two hours, I heard 100 words. The floodgates had opened!

After that, Kurt made fast progress. Video modeling is an evidence-based strategy that worked well for him, so we kept it up. Kurt is now fully conversational and in elementary school without one-on-one support.

After the success with Kurt, I made videos of myself teaching various skills for all my clients. If I was teaching a child to tact, I made videos of me holding up flashcards one at a time while saying the label of each picture. So you might want to take out your phone and make a video of yourself singing a song or tacting items or pictures from your child's materials. Show him the videos, and see what happens.

## Step 1: Start with an Assessment, Plan, and Goal Selection or Revision

Make sure you start with the TAA assessment and planning forms. You'll need these tools to quickly assess your whole child and make a simple plan that you can share with any professionals in his life now or in the near future.

In addition, for most intermediate learners, I recommend standardized language testing administered by an SLP. This was the main recommendation I gave to Drew's family, the three-year-old who liked my yellow racing car. During my assessment when Drew wasn't crying, he was talking in full sentences and using possessives like "Miss Mary's yellow car" and contractions such as "I don't want to," which made his language sound fairly typical. But I'm not trained to administer standardized speech evaluations, and children with more advanced language skills need more testing to determine if they are delayed.

Your child could also benefit from having the VB-MAPP assessment completed, especially if you have a team of professionals and ABA services in place.

Remember: your child's plan and all of his goals need to be based on his assessment results.

## Step 2: Use Your Child's Strengths to Develop More Advanced Language

As I said earlier, if your child is scripting, it isn't an insurmountable problem. In fact, it might even provide you with a way to get more functional language! Continue to look for ways you can use what motivates your child and what he says within his scripting.

If he scripts from movies or loves certain items or activities, for example, you might buy figurines or print pictures of the characters and pair them with the shoebox program. In Lucas's case, I could have gathered pictures of the park or a duck for the shoebox to take advantage of his scripting, "Please do not feed the ducks, quack quack."

You may need to limit the amount of time your child spends stimming and doing things like lining up toys, watching the same videos, looking at the same books, and repeating the same lines. Even if he's talking, he needs to be actively engaged for most of his waking hours. And as he learns more functional language, better social skills, and more age-appropriate leisure activities, his stimming should decrease.

## Step 3: Select Activities and Targets Carefully, and Use Errorless Teaching and Transfer Trials

When selecting activities to build your child's language skills, avoid working on length of utterance, abstract language concepts that are too hard, or pre-academic skills. All skills you teach your child need to be taught errorlessly. All this means is that you provide as much help as your child needs to be successful. For a matching skill, you might provide a point prompt or even a full physical prompt where you guide his hand gently to show your child where to put the identical match. For example, if your child gets confused between "marker" and "crayon," you'd hold up a marker and say "marker" right away to avoid putting him on the spot and prevent an error. This is errorless teaching.

Many years after Lucas was diagnosed and I became an autism professional, I finally learned the secret to preventing and correcting errors, which is one of the critical aspects of the Turn Autism Around approach. This is done through "transfer trials." I even published a peer-reviewed article with my BCBA mentor, Dr. Rick Kubina, about a study I conducted with Lucas using transfer trials to teach tacts errorlessly.[1]

When you use a transfer trial, you transfer a skill from one operant to another, such as going from receptive identification like following directions to touch a body part, to tacting that same body part. For example, you give a direction such as "Touch your nose."

Then once your child touches his nose, you use a transfer trial to attempt to transfer that skill to a tact by saying, "What's this called?" while touching your own nose. Here's another example of a transfer trial: You start with a tact, as the child labels the number three on a flashcard or when you hold up three fingers. Then you transfer that skill to an intraverbal response to the question, "How old are you?" as you eventually fade out the visual of the number three.

You can also use transfer trials to fade your prompts within the same operant. In this situation, you would hold up a picture of a cat and say "cat." After your child responds by also saying "cat," you would move into the transfer trial by saying, "Right! What is it?" If he responds "cat," give him both praise and a reinforcement, such as an edible or a short clip of a movie. If he needs another verbal prompt before he says "cat," provide that prompt, but keep trying to get him to say it more independently when you ask, "What is it?"

Transfer trials enable you to use your child's strengths (like receptive skills) to teach more difficult skills like tacts. Also, using them to fade prompts often improves language and comprehension skills.

As you teach new skills, be careful that your child doesn't develop conditional discrimination errors. This often occurs when they have difficulty discriminating between similar items, such as paper towels and toilet paper or a sofa versus a chair. They aren't making errors because they aren't paying attention. It's just because they don't yet have the receptive language skills for that finer discrimination.

As you can see from this chapter, helping a child expand language skills can be really tricky. It's important to start at the right point (based on the assessment), to use your child's strengths and needs and be on the lookout for language errors that may be halting progress.

In the next few chapters, we'll move on to learning about functional and self-care skills, such as feeding, sleeping, potty training, and making visits to the doctor and the community more successful.

# CHAPTER 10

# Solve Picky Eating

We would all love to have our family sit at the table together and eat healthy food, but in my experience, if a child with autism or delays isn't talking at all or is very delayed with speech, he's likely to have problems with eating. In fact, of the hundreds of young clients I've worked with over the years, I can't think of any who were nonverbal or minimally verbal and didn't also have at least some issue with eating or drinking. One of the reasons for this, of course, is that feeding and talking are intricately related.

Obviously, even typically developing kids struggle with food issues, but it's often worse with children who are delayed. It can lead to problem behaviors because they don't have the language skills to communicate to you what they want. So the language and behavior chapters in this book may also help you solve some of your child's picky eating problems. And if you're struggling to get your child to talk or speak more clearly, this feeding chapter will contain helpful information.

You may think you can solve the issue by ensuring that everyone in the house eats a healthier diet, but that doesn't appear to be true. Years ago, my family participated in a study of hundreds of families conducted by the Milton S. Hershey Medical Center. The researchers learned that even if the parents and siblings ate fruits and vegetables every day, children with autism remained highly selective to carbs, white foods, and crunchy foods.[1] So if you're struggling to get your toddler to eat properly, you're far from alone.

Some children are so picky that they will only eat certain brands, won't eat chipped or broken cookies or crackers, won't eat foods that look or feel a certain way, and will only eat from specific dishes. More recent research by Drs. Susan Mayes and Hana Zickgraf published in 2019 suggests that atypical eating (including severely limited food preferences and refusal of different textured foods) occurs in 70 percent of children with autism which is 15 times more common than in typically developing kids. And in children as young as one, extreme picky eating and other feeding issues can even be a diagnostic indicator for autism as kids on the spectrum are far pickier than children with other developmental delays or disorders.[2]

I have seen 10-year-olds with the same severe eating problems they had when they were young simply because their parents didn't know what to do. So if you're reading this and thinking that you can't tackle your child's food issues right now, I understand. But it will be a whole lot easier to learn and apply this information now when your child is young. An older child is not only bigger, but can become more rigid about eating over time. I've seen a few children with autism who upon entering kindergarten, were still eating baby food and drinking out of a bottle (yet were fully able to chew and swallow corn chips). I've also seen many older kids who never learned how to use utensils and refused to eat all fruits and vegetables. So the sooner you can resolve your child's feeding and drinking issues, the better.

Before we proceed, though, I do need to mention that many children, especially those with autism, have serious feeding issues, including failure to thrive (extremely low weight based on age and height), difficulty chewing and/or swallowing, severe nutritional deficiencies and/or medical issues sometimes requiring tube feeding. Even my son Lucas, at the age of four, was technically classified as "failure to thrive," due at least in part to being an extremely picky eater. We both benefited greatly from attending an intensive feeding clinic at the Children's Hospital of Philadelphia.

So in addition to reading this chapter and finishing the book, if your child has any feeding issues, please consult with a physician, nutritionist, SLP, OT, and/or BCBA with feeding expertise. Explore a feeding clinic at a pediatric teaching hospital if necessary.

There are different feeding approaches and some professionals recommend that children play with food to try to desensitize them to touching foods but not tasting them. But this rarely works. According to Drs. Keith Williams and Laura Seiverling in their book, *Broccoli Boot Camp*, the key to successfully treating selective eating issues is repeated taste exposure. In order for kids to learn to like a particular food, they need to taste that food on 10 to 15 separate occasions. Most parents stop offering foods that are rejected or not eaten readily after on average 1.5 times, thus never getting to the required 10 to 15 tastes. So whether you are trying to improve picky eating on your own or you have a professional helping you, your child has to taste foods repeatedly as part of the feeding improvement plan!

There's a general disclaimer in the front of the book that the information here is for informational purposes only and is not medical or behavioral advice. This is especially important with regard to feeding and drinking information, as only an expert who has evaluated your child can provide direct guidance. If your child isn't growing or gaining weight normally, has difficulty chewing or swallowing, or any serious feeding issue, I recommend getting a professional's help immediately.

## FEEDING ISSUES WITH BILLY AND JACK

Probably my most challenging feeding case through the years was Billy, who would only drink almond milk out of a bottle and eat gluten-free crackers. That's all he consumed morning, noon, and night except for McDonald's French fries on occasion. But he would only eat the fries if they came from the drive-through window and were hot. The fries also needed to be in the "right" container, and he would only eat them if he was really hungry. If the fries weren't exactly as he wanted them, he began to cry and scream. He wasn't getting proper nutrition, so it was a serious problem.

Billy didn't have any language skills, so we started by getting him to respond to table time. Then we used the strategies you'll learn in this chapter to get him to eat a wider variety of foods in order to make sure he wasn't malnourished.

Jack (who was the boy who liked straws from Chapter 6) was another nonverbal toddler with autism who had feeding and drinking issues. He was happy to eat a variety of finger foods (even some vegetables), but when his parents tried to feed him anything mushy from a spoon, he refused. Even the sight of anything mushy caused him distress, so he needed to be desensitized to those kinds of foods and to utensils. We solved this problem by offering him reinforcements (in this case, it was a tablet), while putting one of his favorite finger foods (a corn chip) on a spoon. Then we gradually offered him other foods.

As you learn more about these techniques in this chapter and work on your eating plan, make sure all adults involved with feeding your child are on the same page. Try to keep the same rules and feeding routines at home, daycare, preschool, and the homes of relatives, if possible. For example, if your new rule is that there are no snacks available in between meals and at table time during learning sessions (so your child is truly hungry for meals), make sure his grandmother who babysits twice per week isn't allowing him to graze and eat snacks between meals.

I've found that most parents are able to make great progress using the methods you're about to read. Just don't expect major changes overnight. As with all of the techniques in this book, you will have to exercise great patience.

## ASSESSMENT OF FEEDING ISSUES

As always, the first step in changing the behavior is to do a baseline assessment. You have already done this to some degree with your general Turn Autism Around assessment form, but as soon as correcting feeding problems lands on your plan, you'll most likely need a more detailed and specific assessment related to eating and drinking.

One of the four areas included in Dr. Sundberg's Self-Care Checklist is feeding. I'm including only two levels of the feeding self-care checklist here since I've found the vast majority of my former young clients and children of online participants (regardless if they are 18 months old or 5 years old) are at the 18-month- or 30-month-old level when it comes to feeding.

As you can see from the checklist, most typically developing 18-month-old children can eat finger foods, use a spoon to scoop food, and begin to feed themselves. In addition, most toddlers without delays can drink from open cups and through straws. Using a fork and becoming neater and more independent during meals usually emerges by 30 months. In children with delays and especially in children with autism like Billy and Jack, who like routine and are poor at imitating, skills like drinking out of an open cup or eating from a spoon don't naturally emerge. In many cases, they need to be taught.

Filling out this checklist will help you assess whether or not your child is developmentally delayed with regard to feeding.

---

### FEEDING - BY ABOUT 18 MONTHS

___ Eats finger foods
___ Drinks from a cup by self
___ Uses a spoon to scoop food
___ Sucks from a straw

### FEEDING - BY ABOUT 30 MONTHS

___ Uses a fork to pick up food
___ Uses a napkin to wipe face and hands
___ Carries own lunch box or plate to table
___ Opens own lunch box
___ Opens ziploc bags
___ Uwraps partially opened food packaging
___ Puts a straw into a juice box
___ Takes off own bib

---

## FOOD JOURNALS AND TURN AUTISM AROUND FOOD LIST

Now that you've completed the feeding part of the self-care checklist, I also recommend that you complete a three-day food and drink journal. Using the journal, write down everything your child eats and drinks for three days, including the exact amounts (10 chips, 4 ounces of 2 percent milk), the brands of foods he likes, when he eats, and the location where he eats and drinks throughout the day. This is a baseline assessment like your one-minute baseline videos, so don't introduce new rules or routines, push new foods on your child, or wean the bottle from him during these three days.

Even if you don't introduce any new rules or foods, your child may have some refusal or behavior problems during feeding over the three days. So if he refuses any foods or if any problem behaviors arise during eating, make note of those in your journal as well. Remember to be as specific as possible about any problem behaviors. Instead of writing, "had a tantrum," write down exactly what that tantrum looked like. I'm not a big fan of crying, because, in general, if your child is crying, he is not learning and it often causes stress and disruption to your family. And I'm especially concerned with crying during food consumption. So during the assessment, make note of the foods and drinks your child consumes without a fuss.

Your child didn't become picky overnight, so please don't become stressed about addressing this behavior right away. You won't hurt the situation if he eats junk food and drinks out of a bottle for 72 more hours or even if you wait a few more weeks until you finish this book and complete your feeding assessments.

During your assessment period, you can also use the Turn Autism Around Food List form (also available on the website) in addition to the three-day journal. It includes three lists of foods that I call "easy," "medium," and "difficult." Easy foods are the ones your child will eat consistently without issues. Medium foods are those he has eaten in the past month or two but doesn't eat consistently. Keep in mind that these might include different brands of the same foods on your easy list. Difficult foods are the ones you would like your child to eat, but he fights you when you offer them.

As you can see from Brentley's food list form included here, the easy foods he willingly ate at the time of the assessment included a few fruits, chicken, fries, peanut or sunflower butter and jelly sandwiches, yogurt, "yellow" macaroni and cheese, and a specific kind of oatmeal, as well as lots of junk food. He would sometimes eat eggs, string cheese, a few more fruits, deli turkey meat, and some additional snacks. When Kelsey completed this form, Brentley wouldn't eat any meats besides the chicken strips and turkey deli meat, and he refused all vegetables, potatoes, noodles, and rice.

 **Turn Autism Around Food List Form (Sample)**
by Dr. Mary Barbera

Name: Brentley G.          DOB: 09/25/XX          Date Completed: 10/20/XX

| EASY | MEDIUM | DIFFICULT |
|---|---|---|
| Highly Preferred | Will Eat Sometimes | Will Not Eat |
| Blueberries | Eggs | Sausage (used to be easy) |
| Strawberries | Plain crackers | Meat that is not chicken strips |
| Orange | Banana | Noodles in tomato sauce |
| Mac and cheese (yellow) | Pineapple | Potatoes |
| Fries | Mac and cheese (white) | Any vegetable |
| Chicken strips | Apples | Rice |
| PB and J sandwich | Deli turkey meat | |
| Sunflower butter and J SW | Rice chips | |
| Yogurt | Plain chips | |
| Donuts | Applesauce | |
| Ice cream | Grapes | |
| Candy | Mozzarella string cheese | |
| Chocolate cookies | | |
| Pretzels | | |
| Ritz cheddar crackers | | |
| Goldfish crackers | | |
| Oatmeal with frozen blueberries (only instant apples and cinnamon kind) | | |

Once Kelsey organized Brentley's foods on this form, she was able to see that she had some options to start including a food or two from the medium column during meals. Now, years after his diagnosis and since receiving ABA programming, Kelsey reports that he'll eat any food on his plate, even though he still has his favorites.

Based on completing the feeding self-care checklist, as well as the three-day journal and food list form, the rest of this chapter will help you create your initial feeding plan.

## EXCESSIVE MOUTHING AND PICA

All babies and toddlers tend to mouth objects that aren't edible. Kids with delays, however, sometimes never develop past that stage so that mouthing turns to chewing when their teeth begin to come in.

Sometimes, the reason for this behavior is medical, such as a vitamin or mineral deficiency. Zinc deficiencies in particular may cause excessive mouthing, picky eating, and chewing on toys or their own clothing, while some children may chew excessively because of high lead levels in their system. If your child has excessive mouthing or chewing issues, a medical evaluation with a blood test is warranted, as well as a dental evaluation. But always have a medical consultation before giving your child over-the-counter vitamins or supplements.

Some children chew and swallow inedible objects, which is a serious medical condition called pica. These children may eat coins or liquid soap from the bathroom, or they might pick up mulch and ingest it at the playground. Some children even eat rocks or glass, which can cause bowel perforations among other life-threatening problems. If your child has pica, get immediate medical and behavioral attention.

If your child's mouthing and chewing issues are less severe and medical issues have been ruled out, the cause of the chewing might be to ease the pain of teething. It could also be self-stimulatory behavior, especially if your child hasn't yet transitioned to chewing foods and drinking from an open cup and through a straw.

Assess when and where the chewing and mouthing behavior occurs. If he only does it at a particular playground, stop going to that location, at least for a while. If he chews on his shirt collars or sleeves (and he's already had a blood test and seen a doctor), try shirts with short sleeves or that are more fitted. Loose-fitting shirts might increase chewing.

Some children only mouth and chew when they aren't engaged or when they're hungry. You might try giving him a tablet (as long as he doesn't chew on that) to keep his hands too busy to grab the object he usually chews.

Teaching your child language as you learned about in the last two chapters should also be a major part of the eating plan, as it's hard to mouth, chew on objects, or grind teeth while talking. So the sooner your child learns to speak or use more words, the less he's likely to continue any of these mouthing behaviors.

## DRINKING INTERVENTIONS

Before we talk about strategies for foods, let's talk about how drinking comes into play. As I mentioned earlier, drinking from an open cup and also through a straw are developmental milestones that most 18-month-olds exhibit. These are important for oral motor development, which plays a key role in the ability to form words.

While they may keep your house less messy, spill-proof sippy cups put the lips in an unnatural position that can affect a child's ability to articulate, while straws use different muscles that are important to develop. So if your child is 18 months old or older and still using a sippy cup, one of the first goals in your plan should be to wean him off these. Then he can learn to drink from an open cup and suck liquid through a straw. Even typically developing kids use sippy cups much longer than they should, so as soon as possible, I advise only using a spill-proof sippy cup in the car to avoid spills. Another option is to try spill-proof straw sippy cups for car trips, but the rest of the time, don't make sippy cups available.

Some children with and without delays can have issues weaning from breastfeeding. I breastfed Lucas for more than a year and Spencer for nearly two years. When Lucas was diagnosed, Spencer was about 18 months old, and I was still nursing him. While Lucas loved pacifiers, Spencer didn't. I used to joke that I was Spencer's "human pacifier" because he wanted to nurse constantly.

I was stressed and had my hands full, so I decided to wean him gradually using the pacifier and bottle-weaning techniques included in this chapter. But a few months before Spencer turned two, my husband had the opportunity to take him to Florida to visit his grandparents while I stayed home. Since he was down to nursing a few times per day, I decided we'd go cold turkey for those five days. Some moms continue breastfeeding longer than I did, and while weaning is a personal decision, adding drinking out of open cups and through straws to supplement breastfeeding for children over age one is usually beneficial.

Once your child masters sucking through a straw (which we'll discuss in the weaning section), you can begin to teach him how to drink from an open cup. I've found that small plastic shot glasses are the perfect size to teach young children how far to tilt the cup without spilling. Of course, for safety, use plastic rather than glass, and to avoid a mess during the learning process, fill them only with water. Some families have had success practicing open cup drinking in the bathtub or outside. Sports bottles made for older kids or adults with or without a spout can also be a good choice. You can model drinking from these, and he may imitate you, especially if you're out in the community where he doesn't have other options when he's thirsty.

The biggest piece of advice when it comes to drinking is this: don't allow your child to walk around with easy access to juice or milk (whether dairy or plant milk) in a bottle or sippy cup. I usually recommend allowing only water throughout the day, which will prevent juice spills on your furniture and rugs. Plus, drinks with calories will fill children up, making them less interested in eating nutritious foods at meal time and more resistant to trying new foods. Therefore, if you want to give your child drinks besides water, serve milk, juice, and lemonade only during meals, scheduled snacks, or learning time in a regular cup or a cup with a straw while he is seated at a table.

If your child refuses to drink water and only wants juice or milk, try diluting his favorite beverage with water. On day one, give him one-quarter water and three-quarters juice. On days two and three, give him half water and half juice. On day four, give him three-quarters water and one-quarter juice. On day five, try giving him 100 percent water.

## WEANING OFF BOTTLES AND PACIFIERS

Many children, especially those with behavioral issues, use pacifiers well past infancy. Their parents struggle with what to do about it, so to keep their kids quiet and happy, they just "plug them up" with a pacifier. Lucas was "addicted" to his pacifier well past age two, so I understand.

The same thing can happen with bottles, leaving children addicted to them even beyond the infant stage. In my experience as a BCBA-D, when pacifiers or bottles are given to young children (after the age of one or two especially), they almost always lead to a decrease in language and an increase in articulation issues and problem behaviors.

Over the years, I've also learned that pacifiers and bottles can be detrimental to normal teeth development (both baby and adult teeth). In fact, I had one client who allowed her daughter to continue using pacifiers despite the advice of her speech pathologist. As the child grew older, the pacifier use caused such severe tooth decay and misalignment of her teeth that the dental bills amounted to almost $4,000.

Some families choose the "cold turkey approach" and pick a day to throw away the pacifiers or bottles. But since I don't like kids to cry or stress out a lot, I usually recommend a more gradual weaning approach using the steps below:

1.  Assess when you and your child need the pacifier and/or bottle the most—such as at bedtime, at church, in the car, or while shopping with you.

2.  Using your assessment as your guide, devise a plan with boundaries to gradually wean your child from the bottle or pacifier. For example, "I will only feed him via a bottle four times per day," "He will only have a pacifier prior to bedtime, in the car, and at church," or "I will only give him one bottle at night when I'm at home sitting with him in the rocking chair."

3.  If you use several bottles or pacifiers, hide or dispose of all of them except one or two so that he can't accidentally find one during non-bottle/pacifier times. Keep one pacifier in the bedroom, and if you are going to use one in the car, consider keeping it in the glove compartment where you can maintain control of it.

4.  If you plan to use a pacifier in specific locations or times, such as at bedtime, I recommend you create a "Binky Box" or "Paci Box." After your child awakens, have him place the pacifier in the box when pacifier time is over. Then place the box on a high shelf in the closet. You might need to provide a favorite edible reinforcement or toy. You could say, "Okay, here's our Binky Box. You get a cookie for putting your binky in the box. Then we put that box high up on the shelf." If he asks for a pacifier, cries, or whines, try saying something like, "No, that's just for nap time. You'll get it at nap time. Come on, let's go play with the trains!"

5.  For bottles, give the least preferred drink in the bottle and the most preferred drink in a cup. Pair cups with highly reinforcing toys or edibles during non-bottle times, and keep the bottle out of sight. If he cries or

asks for the bottle, you can say, "No. Bottle is just for nighttime." Once he's calm and not crying, say something like, "Here are your choices." Then offer the cup with his favorite characters, toys, and/or easy edibles. He might have a difficult time for the first day or two, but if you're consistent, he will catch on quickly to the weaning process.

6.  I know it's hard, but don't give your child a pacifier or bottle at the non-designated times, even if he cries for it. No, I don't like crying to go on, but if you provide reinforcement for crying, you will only perpetuate it. Keep bottles and pacifiers out of sight to prevent crying, and offer alternative reinforcements (other cups or even a favorite toy) only when he isn't crying.

7.  At the very minimum, children shouldn't have access to pacifiers or bottles on demand anytime of the day or night. They need you to help them with boundaries!

8.  Over time, reduce pacifier and bottle use more and more until you can wean your child off them entirely.

## FEEDING INTERVENTIONS

First of all, your child should eat all snacks and meals at the dining table. This means no sitting on the sofa eating cereal or grazing on food while walking around. This may be a big transition for you, so your first priority might be to get him to eat most foods at the table. You can do this by giving him only foods from his easy list for meals, snacks, and learning time at the table.

Limit snacks between meals, especially one hour before and one hour after meals. If your child fills up on snacks, he won't be hungry enough at meal times to eat the more nutritious foods you want to introduce into his diet. You need to stop his ability to graze and get any foods he wants throughout the day. Of course, I don't mean to starve your child, but if he's filling up on junk all day, he isn't going to ever want to try new foods.

If your child is under age two, it makes sense to put him in a high chair at the table. But once he reaches two, as long as he doesn't have a physical impairment or severe delay, it's a good idea to begin to transition him from the high chair to a booster seat and eventually to a regular chair. Just as I don't like to trap kids for learning, I also don't like to trap them for eating. If getting your child to eat at the kitchen table becomes a problem, try the same techniques you use to pair the learning table to pair the kitchen table with his highly preferred puzzles and games. Remember that any area, material, person, or location can be paired or re-paired with reinforcement!

Remove foods from their containers so that your child doesn't identify them with packaging or brands. If he will only eat a particular yogurt brand, for example, scoop it out into a bowl. Also, use neutral bowls that don't have any identifying markings. These techniques prevent kids from becoming so specific about what they will and won't eat, so you can then use other brands to expand your child's diet. As a result, he will be much more prepared for eating at a restaurant, daycare, and later at school.

I worked with a boy named Zach who, at age four, was still eating almost nothing but baby food. It was the only way his mother could get fruits, vegetables, and protein into his diet. She was feeding him nearly 50 jars of baby food a week, which was very expensive. To begin to get Zach to eat non–baby foods, his mother started by emptying out the contents into neutral bowls. Once he got used to that, she was able to introduce other items, starting with soft foods that required at least some chewing.

Work on increasing nutrients as much as possible. If your child has any vegetables on his easy list, offer them during all meals and throughout the day when he has a snack. If he has no nutritious foods on his easy list, try providing a vegetable and/or meat from the medium list in between his favorite easy foods, along with reinforcements. If he has no nutritious foods on either his easy or medium lists, you may need to go slower and introduce more medium foods gradually before you can move on to introducing the nutritious foods on the difficult list.

Gradually start presenting medium foods in between the easy foods. Transition first to new foods with a similar look and texture as the easy foods he will eat. Then once you've experienced some success, begin weaving difficult foods into the mix. For example, if he's willing to eat blueberries and yogurt, try introducing blueberry yogurt followed by blueberry pancakes. If he'll eat celery, try to get him to eat zucchini cut into long slices. With Billy, who only drank almond milk and ate gluten-free crackers and McDonald's French fries, we started by making fries at home. Soon, that became one of his easy foods.

If your child is willing to eat soft foods, you can try pureeing meat and vegetables in the beginning. Smoothies can also be a good way to sneak vegetables into his diet, while teaching him at the same time to suck thicker liquids through a straw. But once your child is old enough to chew, you do want him to begin doing that in order to develop those muscles and skills. And as you know by now, this is important for improving both feeding and talking!

During feeding, keep your language positive, short, and sweet. Simply say, "Take a bite." If he eats a less preferred food, offer him a bite of an easy food next. Or perhaps provide some other form of reinforcement like 30 seconds of a favorite video. It may feel like a lot of work to offer reinforcement for every bite of medium (or difficult) food he eats, but it works. Over time, you shouldn't have to offer as much reinforcement as in the beginning.

Avoid negativity, threats, and coercion. Rather than telling him he *can't* have a particular food, tell him he *can* have a different food. Don't bargain with comments like, "Take this one bite, and then you'll get the whole bowl of your favorite noodles." Simply introduce one bite of an easy food, followed by a bite or two of a medium food, and continue back and forth. If he still refuses a medium food, try a different one for the next meal. Keep meals short, and if he refuses to eat, he'll be hungrier for the next meal or snack.

Resist the urge to make your child something special after he refuses even a few bites of a medium food, as this will reinforce his refusal and increase that behavior. Dr. Keith Williams, a BCBA-D and feeding expert who co-authored, *Treating Eating Problems* and *Broccoli Boot Camp*, once said to a young client's mom, "She's no withering flower and will not starve if she misses a meal." That has stuck with me.

If you follow this intervention plan with patience, I think you'll be amazed by how quickly your child will progress.

## TEACHING YOUR CHILD TO USE UTENSILS

While spoon use is expected by 18 months, using a fork and a knife is developmentally appropriate for 30- to 48-month-old children. If your child is significantly delayed, still struggling with severe picky eating, and not getting enough nutritious foods, however, I would solve those problems first. Teaching a child to use utensils independently can wait. It's much more important to make sure he can drink out of an open cup and through a straw and also that he will accept foods off a spoon and fork when you feed him.

When you're ready to add teaching utensils to your plan, I recommend standing behind your child, placing the utensil in his hand, and guiding his hand to scoop food with a spoon or stab with a fork. Once he has mastered using a spoon and fork, move on to a dull knife, and show him how to cut food.

When we were teaching Lucas how to use a knife, there were four of us discussing how to do it. "How do you cut chicken?" we asked, only to discover that we all did it in a different way. I'm right-handed, and one of the other four was left-handed. One adult used the back of the fork, while I used the front. "Should we have him cut up all the chicken or eat one piece at a time?" Who knew teaching a child to cut food could be so complicated?

I recommend teaching your child to cut food the same way you do. If you and your spouse cut it differently, decide on which way you will teach him, and stick to it. (Obviously, if you're left-handed, and your child is right-handed, you may need to make adjustments.)

## EVALUATE, REASSESS, AND MAKE A NEW PLAN

As is the case with every type of behavior, you will need to periodically evaluate how your plan is working. Is your child beginning to eat more foods, particularly nutritious ones? Is he progressing with learning how to use a straw? Are the "medium" foods on his list becoming "easy" ones, and are meal times getting better? If not, do a new assessment to see if anything is different. Then review the strategies in this chapter, followed by a new plan.

Focusing on feeding and improving nutrition is a lifelong goal for many of us and certainly not a once-and-done task. While I think feeding should be among your top priorities, you can't do everything at once.

For you and your child, improving sleep may be a higher priority than tackling feeding issues at this time, so let's move on to that important topic.

# CHAPTER 11

# Stop Playing Musical Beds: Solving Sleep Issues

For a full eight years when Lucas was 2 to 10 years old, most nights we played a game of musical beds. He would take melatonin (an over-the-counter supplement that can aid sleep) before bed, but often, he would awaken in the middle of the night anyway. Once awake, he would leave his bedroom, jump in bed with us, and most times, go back to sleep. If we took him back to his bedroom, he would usually lay awake for hours or become hyperactive. I sometimes sat up with him from 2 A.M. to 5 A.M.

By the time he was 10 years old, Lucas weighed well over 100 pounds, so I began to worry I would become injured when he jumped over me to get to the middle of the bed. I'd be sound asleep, and all of a sudden, 100 pounds of Lucas would come pummeling toward me.

Most nights, we had to choose between staying awake and monitoring him to make sure he stayed in his own bed and was actually sleeping . . . or allowing him to sleep in our bed, where he would often fall asleep quickly. Either way, there wasn't a lot of quality sleep in our house—*for eight years!*

Since I breastfed both of my boys, it wasn't unusual to have one of them in my bed when they were infants. While "co-sleeping" can be controversial and is not recommended, it's quite common. In some families, especially in some cultures, the "family bed" includes the entire family sleeping together for many years.

No matter where infants sleep, most parents go through a period of sleep deprivation when their child is a baby due mostly to nighttime feedings. But we don't expect that period to go on much beyond the six-month or one-year mark when the introduction of solid foods makes nighttime milk feedings unnecessary.

Since my husband worked as a physician and I had two young children 18 months apart, getting each of the boys to sleep through the night in their own beds sounded like a dream (pun intended)! But back in late 1999 when Lucas was diagnosed and Spencer was still breastfeeding around the clock, I had no idea how to achieve that goal. This is why I struggled and didn't sleep through the night for eight years unless I went on a trip. I often say that I traveled to autism conferences not only to learn how to help Lucas but also to sleep alone in a hotel bed peacefully through the night.

If your child has autism or other developmental delays, you might find that like Lucas, he can't sleep through the night in his own bed at ages three, four, five, and older. In her book, *How to Get Your Child to Go to Sleep and Stay Asleep*, Dr. Kirsten Wirth reveals that sleep disorders are common in all children. In fact, 15 percent to 40 percent of typically developing children will have a sleep disorder at sometime in their life. The rate is much higher for children with special needs, who have sleep disorders at a rate of about 85 percent.

Numerous studies show that lack of proper sleep is serious. It can put us at greater risk of developing immune disorders, diabetes, obesity, heart disease, mood disorders, and other problems, and it can reduce our life expectancy. Children with autism also are more likely to exhibit problem behaviors and learning difficulties when they don't get enough sleep.

If insufficient sleep is allowed to continue, your health, the health of your child, and sometimes the health of others in the household could be compromised, especially if you have more than one child sharing a room. In that case, siblings can also end up dangerously sleep deprived.

If you're a parent trying to deal with your child's diagnosis, tantrums, potty training, safety, language development, social skills, and more, how can you possibly do it all if you're operating on too little sleep? And in the middle of the night, you're no doubt so desperate that you'll try anything, even if it ends up making the situation worse in the long run—like allowing your child to sleep in bed with you for months (or years) or taking your child for "sleepy drives."

So sleep problems are often their own kind of emergency that need to be addressed as soon as a child is old enough to sleep on his own.

During those early years with Lucas, I took on most of the responsibility for his sleep issues. After all, I wasn't working outside the home, and my husband was an emergency physician. His job required that he be well rested, or the lives of his patients could be at risk.

Lucas was seven years old when I became a Board Certified Behavior Analyst, but even with my education and experience, I was so sleep deprived that I lacked the clarity or energy to objectively look at his (and by extension, our family's) sleep problems in a way that could solve them.

In fact, when Lucas was 10, I was writing *The Verbal Behavior Approach,* and my husband said to me, "Whatever you do, don't put any advice about sleep in your book because we haven't been able to solve Lucas's sleep issues." He was absolutely right. You won't find a single piece of advice about sleep in that book because I wasn't in a position to offer any.

Shortly after the book came out in 2007, though, I had an experience that started me down a better path. On a trip to Ohio to present a one-day workshop, I had dinner with a fellow behavior analyst. I told her about Lucas's language and behavior—the things I knew well.

Then she asked about sleep. I readily admitted that it had been a real challenge for us. It turned out she specialized in sleep! After telling her about Lucas's sleep patterns and the methods we had tried, she told me she didn't approve of any of them. No big surprise.

She made some concrete recommendations: (1) don't let Lucas get into our bed; (2) keep our bedroom door locked; (3) walk him back to his room as soon as he tries to come into ours; and (4) don't allow him to have a TV in his room (even though it initially helped him fall asleep).

When I got back home, I made a plan to try most of her strategies. First, I explained to Lucas, "I'm going to lock my bedroom door at night, and you need to stay in your own bed through the night. If you do, you'll get a special cookie treat in the morning." He probably wasn't able to fully understand everything I said in that moment, but as we practiced it the first night, it didn't take him long to get the picture.

The first night, he got out of his bed three times, rattled the handle of my locked door, and knocked. So three times, I unlocked my bedroom door, took him back to his bed, reminded him that he would get a cookie in the morning when he woke up in his own bed, kissed him good night, walked back to my bedroom, locked the door again, and went back to sleep. I also looked at the clock and jotted down the times of his knocks, as well as the fact that he didn't engage in any challenging behaviors when escorted back to his room.

The second night, he came to my room twice. The third night, he knocked only once. After that, he never came to my room again in the middle of the night. After eight years of struggling with sleep, this simple intervention corrected the problems for us all in just three nights! I kicked myself for letting it go on for so long.

Since that time with Lucas, I have gone on to work with so many families and parents with young children to resolve a wide variety of sleep issues.

## DEVELOP YOUR OWN SLEEP INTERVENTION

Again, it all starts with the assessment. Of course, if you're sleep deprived, I realize that another assessment may be the last thing you want to do, but it's the first step to getting out of the too-little-sleep cycle. The assessments you've been doing as you've read through the chapters will help you to some degree. If your child has tantrums at bath time or bedtime, for example, your assessment and interventions based on what you learned in the chapter on tantrums will help you with sleep issues. But it's important to understand what happens specifically during your bedtime routine, as any one of these factors could impact your child's ability to sleep.

Below is a list of questions to ask yourself about your child's sleep habits. Be sure to write down your answers on paper or on a device. (Get the forms at TurnAutismAround.com.)

You will need to keep track of progress in order to see important patterns, as well as improvement.

## SLEEP ASSESSMENT QUESTIONS

1. How much total sleep does your child get on average during a 24-hour period?___
   Overnight: Falls asleep: ___
   Wakes for the day: ___
   Naps (if applicable): Start time: ___    End time: ___

2. Describe where your child sleeps:
   Is the room safe (furniture won't fall, blinds without cords, windows secured, etc.)?
   Does your child sleep in a crib, twin bed, and/or share a room or bed?
   If he naps, where do these occur?

3. What does your child's current bedtime routine include?
   Does he eat a snack or take medication or supplements before bed?
   Does he get a shower or bath, brush his teeth, and/or go potty before bed?
   Does he use a pacifier, special stuffed animal, or blanket at night?
   Does he use a tablet, listen to music, or watch TV

before bed?
Do you read books or lie/sit in your child's bed until he falls asleep?
Does your child fall asleep on the couch and do you carry him to his bed?

4. Describe your child's sleep issues:
   How long does it usually take for your child to fall asleep?
   What happens when your child wakes up during the night?

## CREATE YOUR SLEEP PLAN

If your goal is to have your child sleep through the night in his own bed, the only way to accomplish that is to establish a new bedtime routine once your full assessment is complete. If possible, I recommend that one parent take the lead when implementing the initial sleep plan. Once your child is successful over a few nights or few weeks, it's imperative that all your child's caretakers are trained to follow the order of the bedtime routine and are willing and able to carry it out. Your plan will require some trial and error, of course, until you settle on what works.

Here are some recommendations:

**Ensure safety, first and foremost.** It's vital to make sure your child can't leave the house, cause injury to himself or others, or cause property damage. This may require taking all the furniture out of his bedroom so that he can't climb on any pieces or drawers that could fall on him, bolting furniture to the wall (a good idea for all bedrooms), and/or leaving only a mattress on the floor until he learns to sleep through the night. I know this might sound harsh, but sleep is important for both you and your child, so you must take whatever steps are necessary to ensure both safety and sound sleep.

**Transition from crib to bed, when necessary.** If your child sleeps well in his crib, there's rarely a reason to move him to a bed until age three unless he has begun to climb out of the crib. Once he's potty trained, a bed is preferable so that he can walk himself to the bathroom during the night. When you do transition from the crib to the bed, make it a fun event. Take him shopping for the bed, new sheets, and perhaps a new stuffed animal or blanket.

**Stop or decrease naps.** Most children are able to eliminate their morning nap by age two, and afternoon naps can be stopped between ages three and six. Some kids (with and without autism) don't sleep well if they nap at all, however. If your child does take an afternoon nap, make sure it ends by 3 P.M. at the latest. If he falls asleep at 3 P.M. and naps until 5 P.M., he's more likely to have problems falling asleep at 8 P.M. or 9 P.M. Also, limit naps to 60 to 90 minutes or even shorter. Pediatricians generally recommend 12 to 14 total hours of sleep per 24-hour period for children ages one to three. At three, most children can begin to reduce total sleep time to 10 to 12 hours of sleep (including any naps).

You might be thinking that nap time is your *only* break. Also, if your child goes to daycare, napping is usually a required activity for babies through preschoolers. In either of these cases, switching nap time to "quiet time" may be a great option. In order to make this work, you'll need to make sure your child's bedroom is safe, and select quiet toys and books for your child to play with quietly during a set time. I suggest keeping the toys and books in a bin, and rotate these quiet time materials so that they remain special and not accessed at other times.

**Consider weaning your child from the bottle and pacifier, especially if they interfere with sleep.** In the last chapter on feeding, we discussed many reasons why use of bottles and pacifiers past infancy is problematic, and I gave you some ideas on how to wean your child from these habits. If bottles or pacifiers are interfering with your child's sleep or yours, you have one more reason to seriously consider weaning. Most children can be weaned off the bottle by age one, and many parents have found it more difficult to break this habit if they allow it to continue much past age one. Bottles of milk or juice can lead to tooth decay in babies or older children, particularly for those who fall asleep with a bottle in their mouth. The liquid pools and harms their teeth. And if your child wakes up in the middle of the night to an empty bottle, he may want another one in order to fall asleep. Weaning of night feedings will be necessary at some point whether or not your child has autism.

As mentioned in the feeding chapter, pacifier use can also cause tooth and mouth problems if the habit continues for too long. A special blanket or stuffed animal at bedtime can help to replace the bottle or pacifier. Then if your child awakens in the middle of the night, the item he used to soothe himself to sleep is still there to help him doze off again.

**Alter eating habits and avoid stimulants.** You may want to limit liquid intake after dinner, and avoid feeding your child spicy or fatty foods, as well as any foods that tend to upset his stomach. Don't give him multivitamin supplements in the afternoon and evening. Since we're focusing on young children here, caffeine should be avoided altogether, and avoiding sweets and food dyes can also make a big difference.

**Establish your child's bedroom as a place for sleep.** It should not be the place for running around the room, wrestling with a parent or sibling, tickling, watching TV, or playing with toys or a device like a tablet. Put toys and books away in the bedroom or in a different room if your child is prone to getting up in the middle of the night to play, especially if the toys and books could cause injury during the night. If there is no TV currently in the room, and you don't already allow electronics in bed, I highly recommend not introducing them. If, like Lucas, your child already has a TV in his room that helps him fall asleep, you might want to leave it there, at least temporarily. At least with the TV, you can take the remote and have some control over access to it, as well as put it on a sleep timer. Other handheld devices with a screen light are known to cause sleep problems and are more difficult to control/turn off automatically. Like a TV, though, if a tablet or other electronic is already part of the bedtime routine, it might have to be weaned away gradually.

**Avoid the kitchen and family room at bedtime.** Once your child is in the bathroom or bedroom area of the home, it's important to prevent him from returning to the family room or the kitchen for snacks or electronics. You might have to get a gate for your child's room, the top of the stairs, and/or lock your bedroom door like I did with Lucas.

**Avoid getting in bed with your child.** Once you establish yourself as part of the routine, it will be harder to change. If you're already getting in bed with him, you might need to switch to sitting on the edge of the bed or in a chair next to the bed. If necessary, you can lie down on a cot or blowup mattress within the room until he can handle you leaving him there alone. If you want to sleep in your own room, just make sure you continue working toward him sleeping alone.

**Avoid letting your child fall asleep on the couch in the living room.** If you've gotten into the habit of carrying your child to his bed after he falls asleep in a common room, it's a good idea to develop a plan to get out of that habit. Before long, he will be too heavy for you to carry! Plus, if he wakes up in the middle of the night in his bed rather than on the couch, he might struggle to get back to sleep because he's in a different environment. It's best to start bedtime and wake up in the same environment.

**Use gates to keep your child safe.** You may need to have a gate in place at the top of the stairs or in your child's bedroom doorway to prevent him from leaving his room or wandering downstairs if he tends to wake up during the night. For younger children who aren't potty trained, I usually recommend gating their room. For older children who may need to use the bathroom during the night, I recommend gating the top of stairs or other parts of the house.

**Change diapers during the night if he isn't potty trained.** It's important to keep kids clean and dry, so if your child is wet or soiled when he wakes during the night, I would change his diaper and this can prevent irritation and might also help him get back to sleep. If wetting through his diapers seems to be a nightly issue, you might need to limit liquids before bedtime and use the strategies you'll learn in the next chapter on potty training.

**Look into melatonin.** If you've created a good bedtime routine, but your child still struggles to fall asleep, you could speak to your doctor about a supplement such as melatonin. Melatonin is a natural hormone produced in the body, and research indicates that children with autism may not produce enough. Be extra careful about dosage, and know that the long-term effects of this supplement are unknown. The developmental pediatrician who diagnosed Lucas in 1999 recommended we try it because of Lucas's extreme sleep problems early on. Many of my clients also take melatonin—but note that it can backfire for some children, causing bad dreams and an increase in nighttime waking.

**React calmly and consistently when your child wakes up during the night.** Whether he cries, walks through the gate, or knocks on your door, calmly walk him back to his room, saying something like, "Oh, you're awake. Let's get you back in your bed. Good night." You might also want to mention the reinforcement in the morning for sleeping in his bed by adding, "Remember: if you sleep in your bed by yourself, you get a cookie [or whatever reinforcement you've chosen] in the morning."

Only stay in the room briefly unless, given your child's behavior, it's important to stay in the room until he falls back asleep. Some children will need you to sit on the side of the bed or in a rocking chair or even lie down on a blowup mattress on the floor until they are calm and back to sleep. Resist the urge to lie down in the bed with your child if your goal is to get him to sleep through the night in his own bed.

## YOUR BEDTIME ROUTINE CHECKLIST

Your bedtime routine checklist will include all your tasks, as well as your child's tasks, and will need to be completed every night as you prepare for bedtime. First, you have to make some decisions in order to create your plan and new routine.

**Decide on reinforcement.** Like the cookie I offered Lucas if he stayed in his own bed, your plan should include reinforcement. It should be part of your checklist, and you need to decide how and when you will deliver the reinforcement.

Always give praise, but in addition, you can offer edible treats or access to an electronic device in the morning for good sleeping behavior. For kids with more language comprehension, a sticker chart might also work where earning stickers each morning could result in a trip to the store or an inexpensive toy at the end of the week. Based on what you know about your child, try different reinforcements until you find the one that works. The promise of a special cookie in the morning worked well for Lucas, but this might be too long a delay for some kids.

Once you have found a reinforcement that works, *stay consistent* with it. Remember that problem behaviors most often occur when reinforcement is too low and demands are too high. Finding the right balance of reinforcement and demand is critical. If your child is fighting bedtime, try making the bedtime routine a little later to make sure your child is really tired. But consistency is key, so if you try a later routine, give it a good try for about a week. And take data to see if it helps. Remember that bedtime should take minutes, not hours!

Just like we want children "running" to the learning table, we also want kids running (or at least walking calmly) to take a bath, get their pajamas on, and get in bed. If there is screaming or resistance to any part of the bedtime routine, you have work to do. (Some of the strategies in Chapter 13 might help you re-pair these kinds of situations.)

**Establish a leader.** If at all possible, I recommend that one parent or caretaker be in charge of the bedtime routine—at least temporarily until it's well established. It might be convenient for parents to take turns, but this can result in inconsistencies, which can be detrimental to your child's progress. For example, if you usually have your son brush his teeth after putting on his pajamas in the bathroom, but your husband prompts him to brush his teeth before his shower and then to put on his pajamas in the bedroom, this can throw your child off and impact his sleep. If both parents decide to participate in the bedtime routine, it's imperative that all steps of the bedtime routine checklist are followed to the letter in the same order every night. For this reason, be as specific as possible when you write down your bedtime steps.

In addition to the checklist, we implemented a strategy with Lucas that helped both me and Charles, as well as the babysitter, be consistent with the bedtime routine. We got a small photo album marked "Bedtime" and put pictures of the steps in it in order. Then we had Lucas turn the pages so that he and whoever was helping him with the bedtime routine could see and follow the next step in the same order.

In the following example of a bedtime routine checklist, the goal was to get a four-year-old girl with autism to fall asleep and stay asleep through the night without her parents' support or prompting. The parents installed a gate at their daughter's bedroom door, and for the first few nights, they stayed in her room with her until she fell asleep. She now sleeps through the night in her own room.

## SAMPLE BEDTIME ROUTINE CHECKLIST

### Child's Tasks in Order:

- __ Sits on toilet.
- __ Takes bath with assistance.
- __ Puts on pajamas in the bathroom.
- __ Brushes hair.
- __ Brushes teeth with assistance.
- __ Selects three books from the shelf.
- __ Gets into bed.

### Parent's Tasks in Order:

- __ Dims lamp and turns on night light.
- __ Sits on side of bed and reads the three books.
- __ Turns on lullaby music.
- __ Turns off lamp.
- __ Kisses child good night.

\_\_ Reminds child about reinforcement.

\_\_ Puts up gate.

## FIXING MAX'S BEDTIME ROUTINE

When I started consulting with two-year-old Max, he was out of control, not talking, addicted to his bottle, and having huge tantrums many times a day. Yet he wasn't diagnosed with autism.

After working with him for about four months, he turned a corner and avoided the diagnosis altogether, although he still needed some consultation and professional help until he was five.

Max had so many issues in the beginning that I don't think his mom told me about their sleep struggles until he was past age three. But one day, she was so exhausted that the subject came up.

Max had an older sister who was in first grade, and Max attended preschool in the mornings three days per week. He napped in the afternoons and never slept well at night. But he didn't nap in his bed and instead insisted that his mom snuggle with him on the sofa, where he "needed" to rub her thumb to fall asleep for naps. He would then sleep for an hour or two, but his mom was held hostage on the sofa until she had to wake him so she could pick up his sister from school. Naps were clearly a disaster, but bedtime was even worse!

Max never fell asleep in his own bed or slept through the night alone. He wanted to lie down on the sofa and watch TV in the family room to help him fall asleep. Then one of his parents (usually his dad) carried Max to his own room. Even though he was only three, he weighed almost 50 pounds and was especially heavy to carry while sleeping, particularly for his petite mom. Sometimes, Max would wake up immediately while he was being carried, and when he did, it was tempting to lie down in bed with him until he fell asleep again. Most nights, he'd either wake up in the middle of the night and climb into his parents' bed, or one of them would lie down with him and invariably fall asleep there. Like our family, they played musical beds for years.

To solve Max's sleep issues and to help the whole family, we started with an assessment of his nap and bedtime routines (you'll find examples later in the chapter). Max was addicted to his bottle until he was two and a half, so we tackled that to eliminate his need to have a bottle and fall asleep with it.

During the assessment, I learned that after their baths, Max and his sister returned to the kitchen for a snack and to the family room to watch TV. As I explained to his parents, once you take a bath, brush teeth, and put on pajamas, the next and last step should be to lie down in the bed. This prevents watching TV, falling asleep on the sofa, and the need to be carried upstairs. While it may not seem like a big deal to carry a 30- or 50-pound child from the sofa to a bed, it can be unsafe and soon will become impossible.

Max also needed to be tired at night, so naps were shortened and then eliminated. Once Max and his sister were in their separate rooms, I instructed his mom to go back and forth between them. She would read Max a book or two and tell him she would be back in a few minutes after tucking in his sister and reading to her. This enabled Max to stay quiet in bed, as he waited for his mother's return. By that time, he was usually asleep.

Max wasn't potty trained at three, so they gated the bedroom door and responded if he awoke in the middle of the night, changing his diaper if needed and helping him back to bed. Max's mom stopped lying down in his bed and reminded him about the treat he'd get in the morning for sleeping by himself in his own bed.

It took only one or two weeks for Max to settle into the new routine, and the whole family got a lot more sleep!

## GATHER YOUR DATA

In addition to or instead of the bedtime routine checklist, you could use the dedicated calendar that we discussed in Chapter 6 to keep your sleep data. You may need both in the beginning; or if your child responds quickly like Max, you might be able to just jot down his nap and nighttime data on the calendar. Keeping some simple data will help you see what's working and what isn't. You'll keep track of which tasks your child has been able to accomplish

# Turn Autism Around Bedtime Routine Form
## by Dr. Mary Barbera

**Name:** Susie (SC)  **Age:** 4

**Goal:** To fall asleep and sleep through the night without parent support or prompting.

**Key:**  I - Independently  V - Verbal Prompt  M - Modeled Prompt
PP - Partial Physical Prompt  F - Full Physical Guidance

| Bedtime Data | Mon. 5/1 | Tues. 5/2 | Wed. 5/3 | Thur. 5/4 | Fri. 5/5 | Sat. 5/6 | Sun. 5/7 |
|---|---|---|---|---|---|---|---|
| Child tasks: | | | | | | | |
| 1. Sits on toilet | I | | | | | | |
| 2. Takes bath | PP | | | | | | |
| 3. Puts on pajamas in bathroom | F | | | | | | |
| 4. Brushes hair | M | | | | | | |
| 5. Brushes teeth | M | | | | | | |
| 6. Selects three books from shelf | V | | | | | | |
| 7. Gets into bed | I | | | | | | |
| Time medication given | 7:30 | | | | | | |
| Amount of medication dosage | X mg | | | | | | |
| Bedtime | 8:00 | | | | | | |
| After parent tasks are completed: | | | | | | | |
| Time: falls asleep | 8:20 | | | | | | |
| Time: wakes up | 10:40 to 11:05 | | | | | | |
| Time: morning wake up | 6:30 | | | | | | |

Notes:

Gate at bedroom door.
Parent stays in room in chair until SC falls asleep.

successfully and the times that each took place, including what time your child went to sleep and what time he woke up (if he did) and fell back to sleep. You'll also make note of the amount of prompting your child needed to perform each task.

While you're establishing a new bedtime routine, make sure to record whether your child receives any sleep supplements or medications (including the dosage), time and duration of naps, if and when he awakens during the night, what he does while awake during the night, whether any problem behaviors occur during the nighttime waking, and anything else you feel is important.

The more detailed your notes, the better. All of this will help you and any professionals you consult with not only make necessary adjustments to your sleep plan, but also monitor your child's improvement.

For example, you may determine that he gets too excited if he watches television right before bed. You might have to turn the TV off sooner or get rid of electronics altogether at bedtime, replacing them with something more calming like reading three books before bed. You may find that a later bedtime or the elimination of a snack before bath time is better for your child. Each child is unique, so keep up your detective work until you figure out what to do.

Most importantly, always keep your eye on the ultimate goal— your child sleeping through the night in his own bed. Never underestimate the importance of sleep for the health and sanity of everyone in the family. Get professional help if needed, and don't give up until you find the plan that works for you and your child.

I hope you are starting to see how all of these areas overlap, such as how pacifiers can affect talking, feeding, and sleeping. In Chapter 12, we'll move on to another issue many families struggle with and that can affect sleep—potty training. Unless your child is fully potty trained during the day and night, as well as independent with the entire bathroom routine, including handwashing and wiping, you won't want to skip this one.

# CHAPTER 12

# Dispose of the Diapers

Almost all typically developing kids are potty trained by age five, but this is often not the case for children with autism or other developmental delays. I once surveyed parents, and the results showed that only 50 percent of children with autism diagnoses were potty trained by age five. And many children who had been trained were still reliant on a potty schedule, while others still struggled with wiping and bed-wetting.

You may be wondering when you should start potty training and if the typical prerequisites hold true for a child who is delayed. There may be pressure from your child's daycare or preschool to get him fully trained or risk losing his spot in the next classroom. Maybe your child has GI issues with diarrhea and/or constipation, which make it all even more complicated.

Parents of hard-to-potty-train kids (including children with ASD) report all sorts of difficulties. Their child might refuse to go in a bathroom unless it's familiar. He might take off all of his clothing before pooping. He might hold a bowel movement for days until he's constipated, or he may fear sitting on the toilet.

When a child isn't potty trained by the customary age, families suffer a significant loss of time, energy, and resources. It affects their ability to get a babysitter, go to a pool, fly on a plane, visit a restaurant, participate in social activities, and be mainstreamed into the least restrictive school environment. It can interfere with social acceptance, even if the child is unaware of the social stigma of a bowel movement in a diaper, and it can cause discomfort or even embarrassment for everyone in the family, especially if there are siblings involved. I can honestly say that Lucas's toileting accidents when he was around the age of five were among the most stressful and embarrassing times of my life.

Then there's the high cost of diapers for an extended period, not to mention the difficulty of finding diapers big enough for an older child. There might even be additional costs for daycare, which I only realized when Faith's mom was on the verge of paying a premium for preschool because Faith was still in diapers at three. One parent said of toilet training: "This was the most difficult yet most important life skill we have ever taught our son."

If your child is three or older, you've probably already tried to tackle potty training without success. It isn't your fault, but these potty training "false starts" have potentially caused your child to now refuse sitting on the toilet. So my goal with this chapter is to help you create a potty-training plan that's as stress-free as possible. Even if you've already tried and all but given up, know that the strategies you're about to read work in almost all cases.

I'll teach you my system so you'll know when and how to start or restart the potty-training process. The key here is that it's never too early to start planning for potty training and pairing the potty, and it's never too late for toilet training success.

## ASSESSMENT: IS YOUR CHILD READY FOR POTTY TRAINING?

If you read instructions for potty training typical toddlers, you'll probably find a list of prerequisites to determine if they're ready. Generally speaking, typically developing children are thought to be ready when they stay dry for two hours, demonstrate discomfort when diapers are soiled, and have regular bowel movements. They also need to follow simple directions, pull their pants up and down, and request to wear underwear and/or use the toilet.

I've found that a child with delays or an autism or ADHD diagnosis may not need to reach these milestones before you can successfully potty train him. You have to decide when to begin the training based on your individual circumstances. The most important prerequisite skill, however, is your ability to deliver the right amount of reinforcement to teach your child to happily sit and learn from you.

First, it's important to consider your child's developmental age rather than just his chronological (or actual) age. If your three-year-old is only meeting developmental milestones for a typical nine-month-old, you will need to set other goals prior to potty training, such as sitting at the learning table with you, following one-step directions, and learning to wash his hands with help. I don't recommend trying to intensively potty train a three-year-old who is developmentally at a one-year-old level or lower.

Your child might be four or five years old with few language skills and still functioning at an 18-month-old level, so as your child ages, potty training can and should become a higher priority. Nevertheless, I'd work on pairing the table and early learner materials discussed throughout the book before starting intensive potty training, even though you might feel that time is of the essence. I've found that if a child isn't happily running to the learning table, he won't run to the potty and may resist it. So again, before proceeding, it's important that you learn how to teach him and determine what kind of reinforcement he needs.

It will help if he's interested in the bathroom and the toilet, and at least cooperative with some self-care skills such as handwashing and dressing. Does he move away or hide to have bowel movements? That means he's aware when he's having BMs rather than just doing it without awareness, as babies do. It's also helpful if he's having regular bowel movements and not soiling his diaper during the night.

Even if your child is under age three, and potty training isn't officially on your plan, it can help to begin to "prime" potty training as early as 12 or 18 months old. You can do this by sitting him on the potty a couple of times a day for a few minutes with a favorite reinforcement. This way, when you begin to actually train him, he will be desensitized to the bathroom and associate sitting on a small potty with good things.

If your child is under two, I don't recommend that you move on to actually expecting him to pee or poop in the potty or move from regular diapers to elasticized waist diapers or underwear. But getting him accustomed to the potty will make training so much easier when the time comes.

When your child has some language skills, especially manding, and he's able to follow some simple instructions during learning table time, I recommend adding potty training to your plan.

Dr. Mark Sundberg's checklist will help you determine if your child's toileting skills are delayed, as well as how close he is to typical milestones as you work on potty and bowel training.

## TOILETING - READINESS SKILLS - BY ABOUT 24 MONTHS

___ Responds to reinforcement
___ Follows simple directions
___ Seems uncomfortable in soiled diapers
___ Remains dry for 2 hours at a time
___ Bowel movements are predictable and regular
___ Pulls pants down
___ Pulls pants up (with assistance)
___ Can sit still for 2 minutes at a time

## TOILETING - BY ABOUT 36 MONTHS

___ Has learned a word, sign, or PECS for toilet (e.g. potty, pee, sign for toilet)
___ Mands to use the toilet
___ Unbuttons, unsnaps, or unzips pants
___ Sits on toilet
___ Urinates on toilet
___ Wipes after urinating (girls)
___ Defecates on toilet
___ Wipes after defecating (with assistance)
___ Pulls underwear up
___ Pulls pants up
___ Zips, snaps, or buttons pants (with assistance)
___ Flushes toilet
___ Washes hands (with assistance)
___ Dries hands

## TOILETING - BY ABOUT 48 MONTHS

___ Aims into the toilet while standing (boys)
___ Wipes self (girls wipe from front to back)
___ Zips front zippers
___ Buttons front buttons
___ Snaps front snaps
___ Washes and dries hands as part of the toileting routine
___ Nighttime trained (may still have accidents)

As you can see, typically developing children start urinating on the potty first. Bowel movements and then nighttime training usually come later.

## YOUR ASSESSMENT DATA SYSTEM

You can use the TAA potty training form available at Turn AutismAround.com to keep track of what happens each time you attempt potty training. Write down the day and time of each urination (pee) and defecation (poop) and whether it occurred in a regular diaper, an elasticized waist diaper, underwear, or in a toilet/potty. Once your child is wearing underwear, you may be able to scale down data and just write down any accidents that occur within the calendar data system we discussed earlier in the book.

Most of us have patterns, and knowing your child's can help you evaluate and adjust your interventions. The most common times people tend to have bowel movements, for example, are shortly after getting up in the morning and within 30 minutes of eating a meal. This may or may not be true of your child, especially if he has digestive or feeding issues. But if he is consistently pooping after dinner, you will want to take advantage of that when you move from potty training into bowel training.

Children should be having a bowel movement one or two times a day. If it's regularly more or less than that, you may want to evaluate his diet or have him checked by a doctor for any medical issues. I also recommend a book by pediatric urologist Dr. Steve Hodges called *It's No Accident*. He found that 90 percent of the typically developing children who came to his clinic for bed-wetting were actually chronically constipated and impacted due to their diet. Impaction and holding of stool can cause daytime accidents, too. These issues can be even more common in kids with delays because they so often refuse to eat enough fibrous foods like fruits and vegetables.

The one caveat about Dr. Hodges's book is that he recommends a laxative that many parents have reported is problematic. Of course, you should have your child evaluated and check with a doctor before giving him any supplements or medications.

## CREATING YOUR POTTY-TRAINING PLAN

When you put potty training on your plan, make sure you have at least two weeks to be home a lot and work on these skills with your child. The next three months should not include any big changes in the life of your family, such as starting a new school, undergoing surgery, having another child, or moving to a new home.

As you devise your detailed potty-training plan, you may need to start with pairing the potty and/or the bathroom.

## PAIRING THE POTTY AND THE BATHROOM

The first goal is to pair the bathroom and potty with positive reinforcement and make the environment as soothing and inviting as possible. You may need to gradually desensitize your child to his aversion to the room. We'll discuss desensitization more in the next chapter, but for now, consider some unique challenges with toileting. Bathrooms are usually small and enclosed with hard objects and echoing sounds. Then there's the loud sound the toilet makes when it flushes. If your child particularly hates the bathroom, you'll want him to learn how to feel comfortable there so that you can transition him from a small potty to the regular toilet and eventually take him to bathrooms outside the home.

Desensitization may mean having him sit fully clothed on the toilet with a strong reinforcement like a tablet. Then you can slowly transition him to sitting on the seat wearing just his diaper, followed by sitting without the diaper. Throughout this process, you will gradually and systematically re-pair the bathroom and the toileting routine. Your goal is for him to be happy to run to the bathroom—or at least go there without a fight.

## THE WORDS YOU USE

Choose the words you will use, such as potty versus toilet, pee pee versus urinate, or poo or poop versus BM. Write your choices in your plan. Then stay consistent so that your child will not become confused, and make sure anyone who might take him to the bathroom uses the same words and follows the plan.

## THE SCHEDULE

Create a schedule and decide how often you will take your child to the potty. In the beginning, I recommend sitting him on the potty one to two times an hour—set a timer for either 30- or 60-minute intervals. When the timer goes off, tell him, "It's time to go to the potty," or "It's time to go to the bathroom" (whichever word you've chosen). Then set a timer for five minutes once he's on the potty. Prompt him to say or sign "potty," which will begin to prime him for requesting to go to the bathroom when he feels the urge. Have him sit on the potty with a favorite toy, electronic, or book for the whole five minutes, if possible.

## MATERIALS AND REINFORCERS

If your child is small, you'll need a child's potty. I recommend one with a built-in pee guard rather than a detachable one, which tends to get in the way. One of my young clients kept peeing over his potty chair and onto the floor, so his parents got a ring that allowed him to sit on the regular toilet, which worked well. You may also need a step stool in that case for resting his feet and lifting his knees. A step stool can help if your child is accustomed to standing or squatting for a bowel movement while in his diaper.

Once you begin the training, it's best to transition your child to diapers that he can pull up and down himself. The ones that change color when the child pees are useful because you can easily tell when he's wet. Most behavior analysts recommend going straight to underwear, but as a mom, a nurse, and a behavior analyst who has specialized in potty training for decades, I usually recommend a more gradual approach. Elasticized waist diapers will avoid big messes and potential embarrassment to you or the child. Of course, if you transition to underwear, you can always avoid messes by putting elasticized waist diapers on top.

You'll need a timer for adhering to your schedule and keeping track of the number of minutes your child sits on the potty. Keep your schedule and data sheets where you can find them easily, preferably on a clipboard during the two weeks, and keep a pen or pencil attached to the clipboard for easy access.

Reinforcements are also needed to increase any skills. Select reinforcers that you'll use in the bathroom and with the potty based on what you've learned about your child's preferences. Choose a couple of these preferred items, and hold them for use only when toileting. I suggest keeping a "potty bag" of reinforcers that your child can choose from after a successful time in the bathroom.

Make sure the reinforcers are tangible and immediately highly motivating for your child, as well as something within your control. Most kids won't respond immediately to stickers or promises of candy to be given even a few minutes later, for example. A simple "Yay!" or "Good job!" is unlikely to be enough either. Some parents find that using a tablet for the child to watch while seated on the potty works well. Then use an additional reinforcer for peeing on the potty, such as bubbles or a small piece of candy. Don't gauge whether a reinforcer is working by whether or not your child smiles or laughs, though. The only way to tell if it's working is if it results in the desired behavior.

Here are some other possible reinforcers besides a tablet, bubbles, and small pieces of candy:

1. Four ounces of juice, a piece of fruit, or an ice pop. If these are reinforcing for your child, they're excellent choices because you can use them to increase his liquid intake. (You'll learn more about liquid consumption in a moment.)

2. Potty time videos and books. Some even come with a doll and its own little potty. These special potty resources can be helpful to demonstrate to your child

what happens in the bathroom. You can also use your own dolls or stuffed animals to demonstrate, as well as books.

3. There are phone apps available that are great for kids with some receptive language abilities. Some of them even allow you to input your child's name, create an image that looks like him with his name on his shirt, and let him watch the image successfully completing the potty process step by step.

4. If you have an older child who is willing to sit on the potty and demonstrate, you can take pictures or videos to show the child being potty trained. (Of course, be careful not to show any private parts in the photos or videos.)

5. Be creative. One child, who loved umbrellas, did well with his parent twirling a small umbrella around in the bathroom as a reinforcement for peeing.

## POTTY-TRAINING INTERVENTIONS

If your child is very young and not ready for an official potty-training program, I usually recommend placing your child on the potty in the morning and right before bed to get him accustomed to sitting there and also to see if he'll pee.

Also, change his diapers more frequently to keep him as dry as possible. This way, he will become accustomed to being dry and will start to feel uncomfortable with a wet diaper. If he's old enough and has the language skills to understand, you can teach him the difference between wet and dry by showing him a wet paper towel versus a dry paper towel. Then when you change his wet diaper, say, "You're very wet." This helps him notice when he's wet and associate it with the potty. Don't smile, laugh, or be playful while you're changing his diaper, however.

Check him every hour or two, making sure he isn't sitting in a wet or soiled diaper. If you don't know if your child wets every two hours or stays dry for two hours, start changing him every two hours or checking his diaper at that frequency.

Provide extra liquids so that you have more practice on the potty and more awareness on the child's part if there is an accident. (Note, however, that I only consider it an accident if the child urinates or defecates in his underwear; it isn't an accident if he's in a regular or elasticized waist diaper.)

I recommend 2 to 4 ounces of water or other drink per hour for a steady consumption of 8 to 10 glasses per day. Make sure it's steady throughout the day rather than a lot of liquid all at once. A child's bladder can't hold too much liquid at a time, and drinking more than 8 to 10 glasses daily could be unhealthy. You also don't want excessive liquid intake to become a part of his routine.

Boys should be taught to sit on the toilet even for peeing. Otherwise, when you move on to bowel training, you will struggle to get him to sit. Once he has mastered bowel training, you can teach him to stand for peeing.

Your child may enjoy watching you dump the urine from his potty chair into the big toilet and flushing it down. This will get him ready for when he graduates to the regular toilet. If he leaves stool in a regular or elasticized waist diaper that isn't runny, take him into the bathroom so that he can watch you drop the stool into the toilet. Say, "Poop [or whatever word you've chosen to call it] goes in the potty. Flush the potty. Bye-bye, poop!" This will begin to show him where the pee and poop are supposed to go.

Initially, you will just offer reinforcements to your child as he sits and tries to pee or poop. Then when he does sit and pee, you'll provide him with more reinforcement. If he sits and poops, he should get a lot more reinforcement. This is what we call *differential reinforcement*, which means we give more reinforcement for more difficult tasks. This is a powerful strategy to teach children any skill.

Until your child is fully trained, it's a good idea to keep him in regular or elasticized waist diapers when he's sleeping. Once he's in underwear during the day, you might opt to put an elasticized waist diaper or waterproof pants on top to prevent accidental messes. Bodily fluids can contain dangerous bacteria, so you want to avoid messes around the house. One of my clients kept a cheap shower curtain liner under her daughter's chair to prevent too much of a mess in the case of accidents. But keeping your child in underwear during waking hours will help him recognize the discomfort of being wet and encourage him to transition to asking to go to the bathroom. If your child resists wearing underwear, try finding a design with his favorite characters.

Don't punish your child if he has an accident or fails to pee or poop in the potty. If he associates the bathroom with negativity, you will only set the training back and prolong the time it takes for success.

Reinforce *any* new behavior rather than hold reinforcements for perfection. If your child goes into the bathroom with his diaper on to have a bowel movement after he has tended to hide behind the couch for a BM in his diaper, you may want to reward this behavior because it's a step in the right direction.

## ENCOURAGE INDEPENDENCE

Encourage your child to become as independent as possible with pulling his own pants down and up, wiping himself, and washing his hands. If he wears pants, use an elastic waist style because buttons, snaps, zippers, and belts are more difficult for young kids to maneuver. Make sure the elastic isn't too tight so that he can easily get his pants up and down. If they're too snug, he won't be able to reach this milestone.

As your child begins to have success, systemically phase out the toileting schedule. If he is on a schedule of sitting on the toilet every 30 minutes for a period of three days with no accidents in his underwear, you might be able to change the schedule to every hour or so. As he has more successes and stays dry between scheduled times on the potty, reduce the schedule to every hour and a half and then to every two hours. Don't go past every two hours, and continue to provide the extra fluids, even if he has a few accidents, until he's able to initiate the need for the bathroom and successfully use it with very few accidents.

Once he starts to request to go to the bathroom with words, the sign, or a picture, you might be able to drop the schedule entirely or significantly reduce it to every three or four hours. Provide reinforcement for using the toilet independently or for asking for the potty, and phase out the reinforcement when he's requesting to go on his own consistently.

What if your child has stopped having accidents but hasn't transitioned to requesting to go to the bathroom? You certainly don't want the schedule or constant reminders to become a habit (except for reminders before going to sleep or going on a ride). In order to be independent, children need to recognize bladder and bowel urges so that they can begin to go to the bathroom on their own.

To help him initiate on his own, try this: Before entering the bathroom or sitting on the potty, stop him briefly and say, "Where do you have to go?" Prompt him to say "bathroom" or "potty," if necessary.

Of course, if you're using a small potty, you'll need to eventually transition your child to the regular toilet.

## BOWEL TRAINING AND WIPING INTERVENTIONS

Since some parents stop using diapers after their children have been bladder trained, bowel training becomes a messier problem. Your best bet is to make sure reinforcement is *very high* for bowel movements on the toilet. So if BM accidents continue after he's been potty trained, first make sure he's getting enough reinforcement with his preferred items.

He may begin to have bowel movements at the same time he urinates on the potty. If he does, provide extra reinforcement and praise.

If your child is resistant to bowel training after he has been potty trained, be sure to increase the reinforcement further. If he requests a diaper because he knows he needs to have a BM, you might say something like this: "Okay, I'll give you a diaper. First, sit for five minutes on the potty. I'm going to set the timer. Here's your tablet. Then I'll give you a diaper." Or you could tell him that he has to stay in the bathroom with his diaper on. "The only place you can poop is in the bathroom." Have him sit on the toilet or squat over it as he poops in his diaper. This will pair the bathroom with bowel movements.

Wiping can also be difficult to teach. As a parent and professional in the field, I know this tends to be a big issue. So be sure to teach wiping at the start of your potty-training process, and teach all steps. Here's one way you can break down the wiping process for kids:

- Get five to six squares of toilet paper and bundle/fold them.
- Wipe from front to back.
- Look at the paper to see if it's clean.
- Toss dirty paper in the toilet.
- Repeat until the paper is clean.
- Flush and wash hands.

Of course, until he's able to do it on his own, guide his hands as he gets the paper, wipes, flushes, and washes his hands. Be patient, and know that it's difficult to teach "wipe until clean" to toddlers or older children with comprehension issues, as these are abstract language concepts. One solution if your child can't discriminate when to be done with wiping is to come up with a routine to have him pull the toilet paper to his knee, rip, fold, then wipe as he counts to three before repeating the process again. This way, he'll be able to become independent during the bathroom routine and be "clean enough" until bath time.

You can help your child learn some wiping skills like pulling the toilet paper and folding it by practicing parts of the wiping process while he's fully clothed and sitting on the potty.

Most experts recommend that girls wipe front to back to avoid *E. coli* bacteria from entering the vagina and/or urethra. Boys don't have these same physical concerns, so it may be easier for them to wipe through their legs and go back to front.

# HANDWASHING INTERVENTIONS

Handwashing is a really important skill for you to teach your child early on before tackling potty training. This skill becomes even more important during potty training, so make it part of the bathroom routine every time.

If your child hasn't learned how to wash his hands independently yet, you can create a plan and teach him. A step stool will help him reach the sink so that you can prompt him from behind and guide his hands through the process. Assess his ability to accomplish each step, and as he becomes more proficient, guide his hands less and less.

Break down the steps of the task, but don't stop and start each step. Teach it in one fluid action. As you recite the directions, use as few words as possible, such as:

- Push up sleeves
- Turn water on
- Wet hands
- Get soap
- Rub hands
- Rinse hands under water
- Turn water off
- Dry hands

Temperature control can be the most difficult part of the process, so he may particularly need your help with that. As we discussed in the safety chapter, you can also adjust the temperature on your hot water heater or install an anti-scald faucet to keep your child safe from burning himself.

Use the same type of bar or liquid soap, and for consistency, keep it in the same place on the sink. If your child is resistant to physical handwashing prompts, it might be best to demonstrate each step. You can also use video modeling, which we discussed in Chapter 9, and make a video of yourself washing your hands, encouraging him to imitate you.

Keep in mind that if your child is going to daycare or preschool, he may need more prompting to wash his hands there since the routine and location of the sink and soap will be different.

## NIGHTTIME TRAINING AND POST-TRAINING ACCIDENTS

Getting through the night clean and dry is a particular challenge for many young children. As you proceed with daytime training, continue to put your child in regular diapers or elasticized waist diapers during the night. If he wakes up dry for five or more nights in a row, try putting him in underwear overnight, keeping in mind that you may have a few accidents, especially in the beginning.

If bed-wetting persists, you might want to consider reducing or eliminating liquids for the two hours before bedtime. If he's thirsty during that time, allow him to have sips of water only.

If he awakens during the night, take him to the bathroom, and take him there again immediately after he gets up in the morning. It also helps to maintain a regular bedtime and waking time, even on the weekends.

Even after your child has successfully been both bladder and bowel trained, occasional accidents can still happen at night or during the day. First, rule out any medical problems, dietary changes, or medication changes as potential culprits. Then provide more reinforcement, and continue to keep data so that you can assess the cause of the problem.

It isn't uncommon for accidents to happen when a child is suddenly in a new environment like preschool or summer camp. His schedule is thrown off, and he isn't accustomed to the bathroom in the new environment. Make sure he will have the opportunity to request the bathroom at the new place, and keep the lines of communication open, especially during transitions to new settings or caregivers.

Potty training is a behavior just like any other behavior. Make a plan that's based on your child's age, ability levels, and needs in all areas. When you do start or restart potty training, stay positive and be patient. By following your plan and keeping some data, you should begin to see success.

In this chapter we discussed the need to desensitize the bathroom or potty for some children who find them aversive. In the next chapter, we'll explore how to desensitize visits to the doctor and dentist, as well as how to get children to take medicine, take a bath, or get their hair cut without problem behaviors.

# CHAPTER 13

# Desensitize Doctor, Dentist, and Haircut Visits

My two-year-old client Max, who we've discussed a few times already, was never diagnosed with autism. But when I started working with him, he hit his mom, screamed, and cried throughout the day. He struggled even more when his mother took him to a store or anywhere in the community.

The family had a formal event coming up, so they decided Max needed a haircut. She asked that I come along to offer advice.

Max's mom drove us to the closest hair salon without making an appointment or trying to find a place that catered to kids (which were our first two mistakes). Max started crying the moment we entered, and we ended up with their newest hairdresser, who looked like a deer in headlights. Max continued to scream, sob, and flail, so the stylist was unable to do a good job. It was a horrible experience for everyone involved.

Visits to hair stylists, doctors, and dentists can be so stressful that even parents of typically developing kids sometimes put them off. But since children with developmental delays or autism tend to have sensory and communication issues, they often struggle more in these situations. Luckily, there are ways you can desensitize these experiences.

*Desensitization* may sound scary, but it's just a fancy term for the pairing or re-pairing of a setting, an activity, or a person with reinforcement so that the child is calm and comfortable in the presence of a previously aversive situation. Giving your child ample opportunity in a comfortable environment to practice the skills he'll need for a haircut, doctor visit, or other activity is key. Any activity, like taking a bath or playing with Mr. Potato Head, can also become "un-paired" and aversive, so the techniques we'll discuss in this chapter will work in a variety of situations.

Sensory issues can manifest in a number of ways. Some kids with autism or delays overreact to visual stimuli, such as an aversion to bright lights, while others overreact to sound and are bothered by noises. Lucas grew up often wearing noise-canceling headphones because loud noises were a problem for him. Some children don't like the way headphones feel, however, so their parents have to pair the headset with a video or something else the child enjoys.

Some kids overreact to touch and are bothered by clothing tags and anything but soft fabrics. Still other kids overreact to the tastes, textures, temperature, and colors of foods.

Whatever your child's challenge, wearing special clothing, wearing headphones all day long, and severely limiting diets for life are not the goal. You want to help your child learn to tolerate more of the typical sensory input he will face every day.

Nevertheless, I don't recommend trying to desensitize a child to every type of visit at the same time. But once one type of procedure has been desensitized, I've found that the next is often less aversive for the child.

In addition to sensory differences, our children with delays also have language deficits and often don't understand *why* they need to take a bath, get their ears checked, or have their teeth cleaned. They may not know if something is going to be painful and can't tell adults when they're scared. Many kids don't do well with delayed reinforcement or care about the sticker or lollipop at the end of a visit.

In the absence of the techniques you'll learn in this chapter, parents and practitioners have traditionally just held young children down and forced them to go through medical procedures such as ear checks and medication administrations. This makes children feel attacked, so they often fight back. It also makes them extra resistant to such visits so that tantrums might spill over to things like nail clipping and receiving eye drops. I now consider restraining children to be unethical, and I don't recommend it unless it's an emergency.

I also know parents who have experienced such trauma that they attempt to cut their child's hair or do other aversive activities while their child sleeps. Before I was a behavior analyst and knew these strategies, I even tried to cut Lucas's nails while he slept. So I get it. But most of these procedures can't be done with your child sleeping. Luckily, learning these desensitization strategies for re-pairing bath time, food aversions, nail clipping, and haircuts—all of which can be practiced frequently at home—can lead to toleration of difficult procedures. They can also improve talking and reduce tantrums.

Children who can ask for their bath water to be warmer or calmly tell you they'd rather the stylist not use the buzzer around their ears during a haircut will be happier, with better communication and lower problem behaviors.

So I don't recommend completing any tasks while your child is sleeping or holding him down for any procedure unless it's an absolute emergency. When that strategy continues over time, parents end up with an older child who needs three or four people to hold him down, and that puts everyone at risk of injury. This is why it's so important that you learn these desensitization procedures now!

## YOUR ASSESSMENT AND PLAN

You're almost to the end of this book, so by now, you hopefully know that the first step to increase or decrease *any* behavior is assessment.

Doing an assessment of an aversive event, procedure, item, or situation will help you figure out what's truly causing the problem behavior—which parts of what activities are intolerable to your child. For example, during doctor visits, does your child freak out upon arrival at the doctor's office, or is he okay until the weight and height check? Or perhaps the tantrum only begins when the doctor enters the room or when your child sees the stethoscope.

If it has been a while since your child's last doctor or dentist visit, you might have to jog your memory to recall when the problem behaviors usually begin. Do your best to pinpoint the places and the steps within the procedures that triggered your child's problem behaviors, as well as the times when these occurred and what the behaviors looked like.

Then create a task analysis. This is a breakdown of the steps involved with any one medical or nonmedical procedure, such as getting a haircut, taking a bath, or going to the doctor's or dentist's office. You will use this breakdown to further assess which parts of the activity are causing the most issues. During the assessment phase, you might want to determine the location of aversive events or activities and the person or people who are usually involved. You can also use the task analysis for planning and desensitization practice sessions. (Find all the electronic forms at TurnAutismAround.com.)

Since you can't tackle every aversive event at the same time, pick the one that's causing you the most stress. Remember that once you get the hang of these desensitization steps, you can apply them to many situations for all your children for the rest of your life. Let's look at a sample task analysis, assessment, plan, and intervention with haircuts.

# MAKING HAIRCUTS BETTER

Most kids need to visit the barber or hairstylist a lot more frequently than the doctor or dentist, so if they struggle with these visits, it can be a huge issue. Your child can be averse to all sorts of things at a hair salon: the scissors, the proximity of the barber, the spraying water, the plastic cape, or itchy hair falling on the back of his neck.

Before you create your plan for visiting the salon or barber, complete a task analysis of the steps your child will need to do to have a successful haircut:

- Enter hair salon
- Child sits in the chair
- Cape is put on child
- Hair is sprayed with water
- Hair is cut with scissors
- Back of neck and sides cut with electric razor
- Hairbrush is used to brush face and neck
- Cape is removed
- Child waits while parent pays
- Exit salon
- Child is given a highly preferred reinforcement

Once you have the steps outlined, you'll need to decide where you will hold your practice haircut sessions in your home and who will give the pretend haircut. For example, the child would enter the pretend salon in the kitchen and sit in a particular chair. Next, you would place a smock over him, use a spray bottle of warm water to wet his hair, and use play scissors or clippers to pretend to cut his hair.

Your ultimate goal might be to get him to sit through the haircut without screaming or crying. But if he has trouble tolerating the smock, your initial goal might be to simply get him to tolerate wearing it for a few more minutes during each practice session.

It may be necessary to work through the steps very slowly. For example, you might just have your child sit in the practice "haircut" chair and have him tolerate the fake cape or towel you clip around him. Then when he does these two steps in the task analysis, offer a reinforcement, such as watching a short clip of a video or eating something he loves. You can then show him child scissors that are either fake or not sharp at all or you can practice spraying warm water on his head. You may want to stop after just two steps until the next day when he's ready for those two steps plus a third one.

One of my friends who owns a hair salon pointed out that room temperature water in a spray bottle is about 70 degrees Fahrenheit, while our body temperature is usually 98.6 degrees. It may feel too cold and startle some kids—as it did with Lucas. So part of our haircut procedure for Lucas is to fill the spray bottle with fresh warm water before spraying his head, which he tolerates much better.

The key is to go slow, make it fun, and stop while you are having success. Of course, if your child needs a medical procedure immediately or in the near future, you won't be able to go through the steps *too* slowly. But you'll have a greater chance of success if you can spend the time to prepare your child gradually.

If you go too far and your child cries, make sure you don't end the session with crying, as that will lead to negative reinforcement. You might need to use the Sh, Label, and Give Procedure discussed in Chapter 6 to stop the crying before you go back and complete the easy steps.

When you get to the point where he can sit through the entire task analysis at home without a problem, I suggest finding a kid-friendly salon, where they might be willing to work with you in this way. Of course, once you find a salon you're comfortable with, it's important to stick with them. Going to a hair salon without an appointment or a plan like we did with Max was not a good idea. You may also need to ensure that your child has the same stylist every time, and it helps to make appointments when the salon is less busy so there are as few sensory stimuli as possible.

Some kids need a lot of desensitization practice, possibly even visiting the salon a few times without getting a haircut. You might have to practice just getting into the door and sitting in the waiting room a few times, followed by going home and receiving reinforcement. Then you can try having him sit in a salon chair and get his hair sprayed with water. See if the hair salon owner would allow you to bring your home supplies to the salon for a practice session with the stylist watching or helping.

One technique that works well for some children with receptive language skills is taking photos of the hair salon that you can show your child before you go there. We created a photo book for Lucas that used his brother Spencer as a model. We showed him the book and said, "You go inside. Michelle's going to be there. You're going to sit in the chair. Next, you'll wear a cape. Michelle will spray warm water on your hair. Then she's going to make your hair shorter."

There are also commercial books that describe the steps of a haircut, or you could try video modeling in which a typically developing sibling, relative, or friend is shown going to the same salon and getting a haircut. Or you can search for videos on YouTube to prepare children for all kinds of activities such as blood draws, going to the doctor, or getting an X-ray.

At the end of each practice session and especially after your child has graduated to actually going to the salon, provide a strong reinforcer immediately afterward. If he likes to go to the playground or eat a special food, pair that reinforcement with getting a haircut.

Remember to keep data of problem behaviors on ABC charts and/or within your child's calendar system so that you can document progress or setbacks with your practice sessions. For one child who had serious medical issues in addition to autism, we'd rate his behavior at the doctor's office on a scale of 1 to 10, with 10 being outstanding, and we'd document the type of doctor. His behavior ranking improved drastically over time.

## TEACHING YOUR CHILD TO TAKE MEDICATION

What if your child needs to take medicine? When Lucas was a baby, we could put flavored liquid medicine directly into his mouth, and since it was a small amount in a dropper, he usually took it without issues. But as he got older, the volume of liquid medicine required for his larger size became a lot more difficult to administer.

Because Lucas was a very picky eater and underweight when he was diagnosed at age three, doctors recommended that we give him multivitamins and supplements every day. Sometimes, when he was ill, we also needed to give him antibiotics or other medications.

Some parents mix medicines in juice, but Lucas never liked juice. And it was impossible to disguise the taste of the vitamins or medicine in water. In addition, using juice is problematic because it can take a child a long time to finish the full glass, which throws off the timing of the dosage. Crushed pills can sometimes settle at the bottom, which makes it impossible to know how much your child has actually ingested.

So with Lucas, we tried crushing pills in applesauce and feeding them to him one spoonful at a time. We followed each spoonful with a preferred edible reinforcement, followed by another spoonful of the applesauce containing the vitamins or medicine. At times, it didn't taste good, though, so Lucas was resistant to it.

When he reached the age of five, I asked another behavior analyst for advice. Since crushing the pills was causing the applesauce to both smell and taste bad, she said our only recourse was to teach our son how to swallow pills.

Usually, pills for toddlers are quite small, so you can try hiding the pill in a preferred soft food such as applesauce and giving them the spoonful to swallow. This worked with Lucas, as the pill slid right down with the applesauce, and he didn't notice.

If your child is okay with swallowing a gulp of water from an open cup, you can start by giving him a piece of rice, orzo pasta, or the smallest bean you can find for him to practice swallowing. (I don't recommend using small mints or candies because they have a strong taste that may prompt the child to chew.) You can try modeling (or video modeling) by taking the rice or bean yourself after saying, "Watch Mom take a big gulp of water!" Then have the child imitate. Next, try a piece of rice, saying, "Watch Mom put this rice on my tongue!" followed by a gulp of water. Then have the child imitate, and offer him a reinforcement afterward.

Of course, if your child has any serious medical issues, swallowing difficulties, or problem behaviors surrounding medication administration, get help from a professional. As stated throughout this book, all of the information I provide is for informational purposes only and should not be considered medical advice.

## DENTIST AND DOCTOR VISITS

Desensitizing dentist and doctor visits or more invasive medical procedures, such as tolerating eye drop administration or blood draws, can be more difficult than haircuts. Allowing your child to watch a video during an exam is often not possible, and you can't always predict what will happen in a doctor visit, nor can you always take your child to the doctor's office to practice. Some procedures also involve pain or discomfort. To the degree that you can, however, create a task analysis, and practice for each doctor or dental visit. For example, if your child is set to get an ear exam, you could find a toy otoscope or an inexpensive real one to conduct a practice exam at home.

Unless the visit is an emergency, your child shouldn't have to endure crying through it. That said, blood draws and injections cause even typically developing kids to cry, so it's difficult to desensitize toddlers completely from those kinds of experiences.

Dentist visits can be especially problematic for kids with autism or delays, and since these exams only happen one to two times a year, it's hard to work on this skill. If your child has already been to the dentist, start your assessment by recalling everything you can about what happened the last time. Did he get upset on the ride there, when he saw the dental office, when the two of you walked in, when they reclined him in the chair, when the dentist came in, or when the dentist put the little mirror in his mouth?

If your child already has a difficult time with tooth brushing, you will need to start with desensitizing him to that activity. Is he most sensitive to the brush or the toothpaste? You could try a different toothpaste or allow him to taste just a drop of it until he gets used to it. You might have to start by just bringing the brush close to him and making a brushing motion outside of his mouth. When you put the brush inside, you may only manage to brush a couple of teeth at first.

Whatever you manage to accomplish, remember to provide strong reinforcement after each practice session, and keep trying to increase the amount of time he will tolerate the brush in his mouth.

You could also show him how you brush your own teeth, or try the book or video strategy so that he can watch someone else brushing their teeth.

Once you're ready to move on to desensitizing your child for what happens at the dentist's office, I highly recommend getting a dental set with a little mirror and a pick instrument for removing plaque from your local pharmacy store or online. You aren't actually going to scrape his teeth, of course, but you can tap his teeth and rub them with the instrument once he can tolerate it (just make sure the instrument isn't sharp). I did this with Lucas. He sat in the recliner in our living room, and I said, "We're going to practice going to the dentist!" I tilted the recliner back and put a tea towel over him to mimic the dental bib.

When your child has been desensitized to the dental experience at home, ask your dentist if you can make an appointment to take him there to sit in one of their examination chairs while you conduct a practice session with him. Again, I recommend you make appointments when fewer people will be there.

As a side note due to my experience as a registered nurse, autism mom, and advocate for children, if your child must get a filling, I recommend ensuring that your child's dentist uses white composite fillings. Silver fillings contain mercury, so white composites are healthier for both children and adults.

Keep in mind that some children and adults with autism and intellectual disability are not able to tolerate invasive dental work. Lucas still sees a pediatric dentist (who also specializes in and accepts adults with special needs), and he requires anesthesia for anything more extensive than a very brief dental check of his teeth.

Continue to evaluate the success or failure of your strategies. Then conduct a reassessment to make adjustments to your plan.

## GENERAL TIPS FOR PAIRING OR RE-PAIRING ANYTHING

Hopefully, you found the task analysis information helpful, but you might be struggling with desensitization issues for minor activities throughout your day. Over the past two decades, I've seen my son and almost all my clients and online participants have issues at some point with nail clipping, eating new foods, drinking out of different cups, getting used to different beds, or changing babysitters. Some children suddenly hate bath time or suddenly find toys or materials like Mr. Potato Head aversive. While we covered tips for pairing throughout the book, I thought it might be helpful to show you how to re-pair bath time or any activity that suddenly triggers your child to cry or engage in other problem behaviors.

Elena (who we discussed in Chapters 8 and 9) was just 26 months old when her mother Michelle started posting in our online community that all of a sudden, she was screaming during bath time. Michelle was stressed out, so she sponge-bathed Elena for days. I asked her if something happened that might have caused the tub to become aversive. Was the water was too hot? Did Elena go into a pool and get splashed? Was she held down for an ear check at the doctor's office? Sure enough, Michelle reported that Elena had been held down the week before for sedation before an MRI. Until I pointed it out, she didn't realize that something like physical restraint for a medical procedure at the hospital could cause bath time to become problematic.

A few weeks later, after following the advice of our online community, Michelle had turned things completely around, and Elena was asking for a bath! "She won't even wait for me to fill the tub before climbing in. And when we're all done, she says 'play some more' because she doesn't want to get out!" Michelle reported.

Here are the strategies Michelle used for re-pairing bath time:

- Play with favorite toys in the tub with *no* water in it, with clothes on, and then gradually with clothes off.

- Gather and consider purchasing new tub toys (fishing pole with magnetic fish, bath crayons, bubble bath, cups to pour water, etc.)

- Fill the tub with warm water, and encourage child to stand outside the tub and reach into the water to play with toys.

- Encourage child to put feet in the water for a few seconds, and allow/help him in the following days to step safely out of the tub whenever he wants.

- Gradually, as the child stands for longer periods and plays with toys, pour water over his feet and belly, and use a sponge to wash.

- Encourage sitting in the tub (may happen naturally as child is playing with tub toys).

The process wasn't perfect, and Michelle reported that there were some problem behaviors like whining. Elena said "no" when her mother pushed her too quickly. But for minor problem behaviors, Michelle would just step back a little and say things like, "We don't have to sit in the tub today, but we'll try again tomorrow." Or she offered Elena some choices, such as, "Should Mommy wash your arms or feet first?"

Hopefully, this information on desensitization and pairing will help you prevent and fix aversive situations that are happening now, as well as those that may come up for your child later. If you take only two things from this chapter, remember these points: (1) Don't hold your child down or allow professionals to restrain him unless it's an emergency. (2) Any person, place, object, procedure, or activity can be paired or re-paired with time, practice, and patience.

It's time to move on to the final chapter where I'll cover how to find professionals, schools, and services that may be part of the solution. We'll also discuss how to settle in to the "captain's seat" so you can advocate for your child and your whole family for life. And I'll summarize the four key steps of the Turn Autism Around approach that you can take right now to help you and your child continue to make great strides for years to come.

# CHAPTER 14

# Become Your Child's Best Teacher and Advocate for Life

I'm so excited that you made it here to the final chapter! I hope you're starting to feel less worried and more confident that you can start turning autism around.

Whether you've read this book in one sitting or have taken your time, I suspect you are already a different person. The questions you may have been asking at the beginning of the book, such as, *Is my child just stubborn or a late talker?* or *Are these signs of ADHD or autism?* may not seem as important anymore.

Indeed, the most important question from the first page of the book is this one: *Is there something I can do to help my child, regardless of the diagnosis?*

And now you know there is a lot you can do!

But you may also have another problem. You might be overwhelmed by so much information—or you have too many strategies to try to implement. You're probably feeling a ton of pressure as the newly appointed "captain of the ship."

You can't solve every problem alone, and you have to take care of yourself and your whole family while you steer the ship and navigate through the rough waters. And you know *time is of the essence*. So, how do you do it all?

## GETTING THE HELP YOU NEED

You can and should use the Turn Autism Around approach throughout your day (and night) to help your child learn new skills. But unless your child only has a minor delay and catches up quickly, you will most likely need help.

While this book and my online programs encourage parents to start engaging their children in 15-minute sessions daily, studies show that young children with autism need at least 20 hours per week of intensive ABA programming, while some children may need up to 40 hours per week.

Even if your child's therapy sessions are not currently ideal, take some deep breaths and try to improve the situation. The professionals in your child's life now or in the future are all good people, many with years of education and experience. Like you, they want your child to succeed. Collaborate with them, and share how the Turn Autism Around approach is helping your child.

Some health care providers, autism professionals, and even family members and friends may warn you that your child is "too high functioning," "too low functioning," "too old," or "too young" to benefit from ABA and the TAA approach. But this isn't true. As long as your child isn't fully conversational and struggles in any area, he can benefit.

I used to always recommend ABA and SLP services for every child with delays, thinking that therapy of any kind delivered by a professional was always better than no therapy. But over the past few years, after working directly with hundreds of children and training thousands of families and professionals from more than 80 countries, I've changed my stance.

For example, Sarah joined my online program to help her son, two-year-old Connor, who had just been diagnosed with autism and was on a waiting list for intensive ABA therapy. Within two weeks, Connor loved table time and said his first word, "apple."

After a few months, Connor's family got to the front of the line for ABA therapy for four hours per day. They were excited to accelerate his learning, but the BCBA from the ABA company warned the family that there would be a lot of crying in the beginning because they would require him to sit at the table and do "work." Plus, the BCBA wasn't interested in reviewing the TAA forms or the videos of Connor's amazing progress in only two months.

Sarah kept encouraging the BCBA to watch the pre- and post-videos she recorded of Connor. She worked with the BCBA to use the early learner activities and materials that Connor was used to so that he wouldn't cry during table time. Her persistence paid off, and she was able to help the staff learn and incorporate the TAA strategies that had been so successful.

But many families are not able to find professionals who are willing to collaborate, at least not right away. And some parents like Kelsey and many others have to walk away from professionals, settings, or programs when it becomes clear that they aren't helping.

As a result, I now believe that *no therapy is better than bad therapy*. So if you struggle at first to find the help you need, you can take comfort because you now know how to engage and teach your child. Therefore, you won't ever have to resort to "no therapy." And while you work with your child at home, you can take some time to find the right professionals who will allow you to remain the captain of the ship and an important member of your child's team.

In addition to professionals, you'll probably need other non-professionals who can keep your child as safe and engaged as possible. While it may seem daunting, all children—especially those with autism—need engagement most of their waking hours, and this equals approximately 100 hours per week. Obviously, you can't do it alone. When my boys were young, I hired "Mommy's helpers," babysitters, and nannies for several years, who provided additional care for Lucas and Spencer while I worked as a behavior analyst, pursued my Ph.D., and wrote my first book. I also enlisted the help of my husband, parents, sister, and friends.

Because of the insurance regulations that funded Lucas's program, someone needed to be in the house while he received 40 hours per week of ABA therapy in the basement. One time when I had an appointment, my dad watched Spencer upstairs while

Lucas was in a therapy session. When I returned home, he joked that it was almost like I was on "house arrest." I know it can feel that way sometimes.

So if you can get assistance from family and friends and/or if you have the funds to hire help, I strongly recommend all of the above. But even if you can afford the best of the best, you'll still need to learn to advocate for quality services and remain a big part of your child's program.

## HIGH FUNCTIONING VERSUS LOW FUNCTIONING

Labels of "high functioning" or "low functioning" are usually too subjective to be helpful. Let's say you're a teacher with six or eight kids with autism in your classroom, and you're asked to line up your students in terms of the highest functioning to the lowest functioning. You'd have a terrible time trying to do that. Are you evaluating them based on problem behaviors? Academics and language? Social abilities?

I've observed parents and professionals who, understandably, want to diminish a child's issues by calling him "high functioning." To the degree a child appears typical, however, the more you'll probably have to advocate for him within the health care and school systems because it may appear as though he doesn't need services. So as tempting as it may be to have your child labeled "high functioning," it's unlikely to change his needs.

While many kids labeled as such can eventually be included in general education settings and may be high enough functioning to learn how to drive, go to college, and perhaps get married, high-functioning autism may also come with some comorbid conditions like a higher rate of anxiety, depression, and other problems.

When people use the term *low functioning*, they're usually describing kids who also have an intellectual disability with little to no language. But there's a whole spectrum in between going to college and driving a car and needing constant support and supervision. Some children labeled high functioning are fully conversational, but they can't hold a job due to anxiety or depression. Others described as low functioning grow up to be gainfully employed and happy, living with only minor support.

The bottom line is to provide your child with as much teaching and therapy as you can regardless of whether you deem his delays or autism diagnosis as "severe" or "mild." Without sufficient intervention, children with mild delays or a mild autism diagnosis can end up with more long-term issues than children with severe delays or a severe diagnosis. You'll never feel like you've given your child too much intervention, but you might someday conclude that you haven't provided enough.

## ADVOCACY FOR LIFE

Advocacy is a lifelong skill. Even for my typically developing son, Spencer, I never stopped learning how to be a better teacher and advocate for him. I've discovered over the years that there is no such thing as being "just a parent" and that being the best parent you can be means taking on the roles of teacher and advocate, too.

Like Sarah, advocating for ABA and for others to use the Turn Autism Around approach may be your next hurdle to jump over. While you may be lucky enough to never have to advocate for your child to receive the services and education he needs, there's a good chance you will have to.

The harsh truth is that even more than two decades after I was thrown into the autism world, most young children with delays and early warning signs of autism still don't receive nearly enough services to make a difference. Very few organizations provide quality ABA programming in homes or at clinics and schools. It's one of the main reasons I was so passionate about writing this book.

So, what if you can't find a BCBA or other autism professional in your area, or you find one who isn't receptive to the Turn Autism Around approach? If you have an unreceptive BCBA, teacher, SLP,

OT, or administrator, I recommend that you share your assessment, plan, language samples, and videos with them to show your success in working with your child at home. If they can see data and video evidence of the success you're achieving, they might change their minds.

You may need to work with your preschool, insurance provider, and/or school district to develop the kinds of programs your child (and other children with delays and autism) need. It will no doubt push you outside your comfort zone, but your child's future is at stake.

Know that regardless of where you live in the world, any agency or organization that is funding your child's therapy will need baseline and ongoing data, a plan, and goals. They will also need to keep track of progress. So you should do the same, even if you are teaching your child yourself at home.

Make it a priority to keep organized and meticulous records of your child's needs, assessments, interventions, progress, and the services he has received to date. Keep all of it in a three-ring binder organized in sections. These documents will be your best ammunition if you need to advocate. Not only will the information be important, but it will also show anyone who sees your well-organized binder that you're serious.

You will also be required to—and should want to—attend meetings to discuss your child's interventions and education. If possible, I recommend that you bring someone supportive with you to each meeting. If you find yourself opposed by a group of people, you'll be grateful to have someone there who's on your side. Also, having this person take notes during the meeting will help if you need to follow up in writing.

Always remember, however: *Advocacy should not be the same as fighting.* It shouldn't be "us against them." Everyone should work together to ensure that each child reaches their fullest potential. It shouldn't be about opinions, either; it should be about how to get your child to the next level based on his strengths and needs, data collected on progress, and your family's priorities.

In some cases, you might even need an independent evaluation or someone outside the current team who can come in to mediate the situation. They may be able to better see where the true disagreement lies and how you might get back on track.

There are, of course, professional advocates, and I recommend you get one if that's an option for you. I was able to find a free advocate from a mental health association in my area, but there are paid advocates and lawyers who can assist you if you have the funds. There may also be advocacy workshops in your area or online where you can learn more.

Meanwhile, get as much support as you can from friends, extended family members, and like-minded professionals. Learn to ask for help, even if it's just to vent your frustrations and worries. If anyone questions your methods, ask them to read this book.

It's also helpful to look for an online or local support group for parents of children with autism or delays. They will be a source of both emotional support and resources. You can learn a great deal from other parents who may have dealt with some of the same issues before you, particularly as it relates to advocacy in your specific area.

There's no clear-cut moment, however, when you can stop advocating for your child because he has reached some proverbial "next level." Just keep putting one foot in front of the other, and stay confident in your abilities to do what's necessary. You're now armed with lots of information that will help you along your journey of advocacy.

## FOUR STEPS OF THE TURN AUTISM AROUND APPROACH

The Turn Autism Around approach includes four steps to take regardless of the problem or what area it falls under. So whether you want to teach your child to talk, reduce crying, teach him to sleep in his own bed, or make visits to the doctor easier, you'll follow the same process. Here is a summary of the four main steps:

1. **Assessment.** The first step to solving any problem is assessment, and the TAA assessment form is the best place to start or to use for reassessment. I know I've hammered this hard throughout the book, but starting with the assessment is truly that important. You can also use any recent medical and therapy evaluations and reports, as well as additional assessments covered throughout this book. After completing and reviewing the assessments, your next step is to compare your child's levels with typical milestones to determine any gaps in his development. (Remember to check out the electronic copies of all forms and resources at TurnAutismAround.com.)

   You or the professionals on your child's team may not think you need to complete the one-page assessment, especially if you already have dozens of pages documenting his development. But before you or any professionals can implement the TAA approach, it's important that you have one page where you can get a quick overview of your child's strengths and needs in multiple areas. This assessment tool gives you a snapshot of possible issues such as pacifier addiction, sleep problems, and inability to use words functionally, among many other areas of development. It isn't possible to effectively implement the TAA approach without this step.

   If there are medical issues, or there are gaps in your child's development that are concerning you, please also speak with your child's physician. You may also need to seek evaluations by an SLP, developmental pediatrician, or other health care providers. Unfortunately, this may involve getting on waiting lists and using some of the advocacy strategies we've discussed.

2. **Planning.** The next step is to complete or update the TAA planning form discussed in Chapter 5. Ensure that any early intervention or ABA plans or goals that may already be in place are based on the TAA assessment, as it's quite common to see a disconnect between the assessment and the plan. For example, someone on an ABA clinic staff might say they use a verbal behavior type of ABA program and complete the VB-MAPP assessment to get insurance authorization for services. But their plan and goals include a heavy focus on improving eye contact, increasing length of utterance, and working on abstract language targets that are way too difficult. So make sure the TAA plan and goals are based on the TAA assessment.

3. **Teaching.** It's important that you keep your child as engaged as possible throughout the day. Be positive and spend 95 percent of your time preventing problem behaviors. Use the TAA plan and goals to select what to work on and what activities and materials to use.

4. **Evaluating Progress.** Collect data on what you're teaching your child and how he is progressing. Modify your daily teaching sessions based on the data you collect. I also recommend you update the assessment and planning forms regularly. The more progress your child makes, the more frequently you must update these forms—perhaps every few months. Use the calendar data system we discussed in Chapter 6 to monitor medical and behavioral issues, and keep ABC data to track major problem behaviors so that you can analyze how to prevent them.

## YOUR CHILD'S HAPPINESS—AND YOUR FAMILY'S HAPPINESS—ARE PARAMOUNT

Children with autism or signs of autism rarely get the intensive early behavioral intervention services they need. Instead, they often receive more like one to three hours of eclectic treatments per week during the most critical time of their development. As the numbers of diagnoses increase, early intervention agencies and school systems are stressed trying to meet the complex and varying needs of children with delays and autism. That's why you, as the parent, have to learn as much as you can and advocate for your child. No one knows him as well as you do, and no one has more motivation to see him succeed.

Our kids simply don't have time to wait. As I said in Chapter 1, the bottom line is that getting ahead of difficult behaviors and catching up with language and social skills is far more significant than the diagnosis. *You can't afford to go into denial (like I did) or play the waiting game.*

But I urge you not to succumb to regret. It's easy to kick yourself if you feel you've made mistakes. This isn't the time to blame yourself for listening to others who told you to "be patient" as you passively waited in line while your child regressed more. It isn't helpful to be angry at your child's doctor or the speech therapist who both gave you false reassurances and said there were no delays when your son was a toddler. And it's not helpful to think about your child's ABA provider who told you a year or two ago that scripting was "just a part" of autism.

I think the chapters you've read in this book have shown you that despite what you may have already gone through or what you might have been told, you have the power to reverse some of the earliest signs of autism. You can teach your child to communicate, potty train him, get him to sleep in his own bed throughout the night, get him to eat meals with your family, and take him to the doctor and barber, regardless of whether or not he ever receives an autism diagnosis.

If your child does have a diagnosis or goes on to get one, however, remember that no one has a crystal ball to know how everything will turn out for your child. It's impossible to predict, for example, how a 2-year-old is going to be at age 8 or age 18. What we *can* predict is that you can improve the quality of your child's life with early and intensive interventions.

Twenty years ago, I thought I could fix everything quickly and get back to a "normal" life. I thought of recovery for Lucas as black and white, and I fantasized about a recovery party for him at some point. But I learned that no one has a "normal" life. And there's certainly no such thing as "perfect."

Your child only has one life, but so do you and so does everyone in your family. It will be a marathon and not a sprint. I often say it will be more like a marathon on a roller coaster with unexpected twists and turns, so don't forget to take care of yourself, too.

You might not believe me yet, but as you step into the role of captain to start to turn autism (or signs of autism) around, you will not only change your child's life in a positive way, but you'll change your life for the better as well.

This is not the kind of book that you'll want to loan out or give away, because chances are, you'll need to reread chapters or sections as your child learns and grows. What you've read may have helped you climb out of a hole you'd fallen into or helped you get a quarter of the way up the mountain. Hopefully, it's less scary now with clearer skies ahead.

But reading this book will never be enough. You'll have to keep climbing the mountain and become a lifelong learner. And I'll continue to be here by your side as your guide. My mission is to Turn Autism Around for millions of families worldwide.

Throughout the climb that Lucas; his typical brother, Spencer; and the rest of my family has made, my goal for both my children has remained unchanged. And that goal is for both of them to be as *safe, independent, and happy as possible* and to reach their fullest potential. That's my goal and greatest hope for all your children, too.

**ABA: Applied Behavior Analysis.** The science of changing socially significant behavior; behavioral programs for children with autism to increase language and learning skills and reduce problem behaviors.

**ADHD: Attention Deficit Hyperactivity Disorder.** A neurodevelopmental disorder, usually characterized by inattention or hyperactivity and impulsive behavior that interferes with learning or development.

**Autism or ASD: Autism Spectrum Disorder.** Developmental disorder with impairment of language and social communication skills, as well as repetitive or restrictive interests. It's a "spectrum" disorder because there is wide variation in types of symptoms, as well as severity.

**BCBA or BCBA-D.** A Board Certified Behavior Analyst has satisfied the education and experience requirements and passed a certification exam. A BCBA holds at least a master's degree, and a BCBA-D holds a doctorate degree.

**Conditional discrimination.** The ability to discriminate between similar things, such as labeling toilet paper versus paper towels or answering "who" versus "where" questions.

**Delayed echolalia.** Repeating words or phrases heard in the past and using these in a script-like fashion. Can also be called "scripting" or "stimming."

**Desensitization.** Pairing or re-pairing a setting, activity, or person with reinforcement so that a child is calm and comfortable when faced with a previously aversive situation.

**Echoic.** Repeating what someone else says. Can be immediate or delayed. One of the four elementary verbal operants as defined by Dr. B. F. Skinner in *Verbal Behavior*.

**Echoic control.** The ability to get a child to repeat words or phrases without an object or picture present. For example, a child says "ball" when you prompt, "Say 'ball.'"

**Errorless teaching.** An instructional strategy to ensure a child always gives the correct response. All mistakes are prevented by providing a prompt immediately after the direction is given or question is asked.

**Expressive language.** Use of gestures, words, and sentences to communicate wants and needs and eventually thoughts and ideas with others. Made up of the four elementary verbal operants (mands, tacts, echoics, and intraverbals).

**Generalization.** To perform a skill under different conditions in a different way with different materials, or to a different person, and to continue to exhibit that skill over time. For example, after learning to label a picture of a cat, the child will say "cat" at the sight of a live cat.

**Hyperlexia.** The ability to read letters and words that is more advanced than would be expected for chronological age or functional language level; intense fascination with letters and numbers.

**Imitation skills.** Copying or mimicking someone else's behavior and movements.

**Intraverbal.** Filling in blanks or answering "WH" questions; responding to someone else's verbal behavior with no visual or other stimuli. One of the four elementary verbal operants as defined by Dr. B. F. Skinner in *Verbal Behavior*.

**Joint attention.** An important social skill that means focusing on the same item or activity with awareness that attention is being shared.

**Mand.** A request for an item, action, attention, or information. Motivation is the antecedent for a mand, and the consequence is direct reinforcement, making the mand the most important of the four elementary verbal operants as defined by Dr. B. F. Skinner in *Verbal Behavior*.

**Matching skills.** The ability to match identical or similar items or pictures.

**M-CHAT: Modified Checklist for Autism in Toddlers.** A validated developmental screening tool for toddlers between 16 and 30 months of age. It is designed to help identify children who may benefit from additional developmental and autism evaluations.

**Multiple control.** Combining two or more operants (mands, tacts, and/or echoics) to improve learning. Multiple control is used extensively in the early learner activities within the Turn Autism Around approach so that if a child says a word, it is part mand, part tact, and part echoic.

**Operant.** A behavior defined in terms of its antecedent and consequence. For example, the antecedent of a mand is motivation, and the consequence of asking for an item is receiving the requested item. The four elementary verbal operants are mand, tact, echoic, and intraverbal.

**OT: Occupational Therapy.** A type of therapy that helps individuals with motor skills involved with everyday life, regulation of sensory processing dysfunctions, and working within teams on activities of daily living, including feeding, grooming, dressing, and potty training.

**Pairing.** The ongoing process of using a child's already established reinforcers (things he likes) to make new people, difficult materials or tasks, and unknown environments more positively reinforcing.

**Pica.** A medical and potentially life-threatening condition in which children eat inedible items such as soap, dirt, rocks, or feces. Pica requires immediate consultation with a health care provider.

**Pop out words.** Words that children say from time to time but will not say upon request.

**Prompt.** A hint or cue to help a child give the correct response. There are several types of prompts, including physical (you gently help the child move through a motion), gestural (you point to the area), imitative (you touch your head while saying "touch head"), and verbal (you add words to clarify or give a reminder).

**Receptive language.** The ability to understand and comprehend spoken language.

**Regression.** The loss of skills or language that children with autism or delays had previously.

**Reinforcement/Reinforcer.** A food, toy, other item, action, or attention, such as praise, that increases the probability that a behavior will increase in the future.

**Scripting.** Repetition of words, phrases, or lines from movies without an understanding of their meaning. Also called "delayed echolalia."

**SIB: Self-Injurious Behavior.** A problem behavior in which a child injures himself, such as repeatedly banging his head with his fist or scratching his body. SIB requires immediate consultation with a health care provider.

**Skinner, B. F.** The founder of the experimental analysis of behavior and the author of the 1957 book *Verbal Behavior*.

**SLP: Speech and Language Pathologist.** A health care professional trained to evaluate and treat people with speech, language, communication, swallowing, or hearing disorders.

**STAT: Screening Tool for Autism in Toddlers.** An interactive screening tool developed by Dr. Wendy Stone that includes a set of 12 activities that measure a child's social communication skills and risk for autism.

**Stimming.** Self-stimulatory behavior that usually involves repetitive movements (hand flapping, rocking, etc.), making sounds (also known as "verbal stimming"), or repeating lines from movies or things heard in the past (also known as "scripting").

**Tact.** Labeling or naming an object, picture, adjective, location, smell, taste, noise, or feeling. One of the four elementary verbal operants as defined by Dr. B. F. Skinner in *Verbal Behavior*.

**Transfer trial.** The process of fading a prompt or transferring a skill from one operant to another, such as going from receptive identification of a body part to tacting of that same body part.

**VB-MAPP: Verbal Behavior Milestones Assessment and Placement Program.** An in-depth assessment and curriculum guide developed by Dr. Mark Sundberg and based on B. F. Skinner's analysis of verbal behavior outlined in the *Verbal Behavior* book.

**Video modeling.** An evidence-based strategy in which a video is made of someone modeling the behavior you want to increase.

# ENDNOTES

## Chapter I

1. Centers for Disease Control and Prevention, "Increase in Developmental Disabilities Among Children in the United States," accessed July 28, 2020, https://www.cdc.gov/ncbddd/developmentaldisabilities/features/increase-in-developmental-disabilities.html.

2. A. Klin and W. Jones, "An Agenda for 21st Century Neurodevelopmental Medicine: Lessons from Autism," *Revista de Neurologia* 66, S01 (March 2018): S3–S15.

3. A. Klin et al., "Affording Autism an Early Brain Development Re-definition," *Development & Psychopathology*, (September 2020): 1–15. https://doi.org/10.1017/S0954579420000802.

4. Ibid; A. Klin, "Recent Advances in Research and Community Solutions Focused on Early Development of Social Responding in Infants and Toddlers with Autism," National Autism Conference, August 3, 2020, https://sched.co/cYfb.

5. O. I. Lovaas, "Behavioral Treatment and Normal Educational and Intellectual Functioning in Young Autistic Children," *Journal of Consulting & Clinical Psychology* 55, (1987): 3–9.

6. M. Sarris, "'Recovery' by the Numbers: How Often Do Children Lose an Autism Diagnosis," Interactive Autism Network at Kennedy Krieger Network, last modified January 27, 2016, https://iancommunity.org/ssc/recovery-numbers-how-often-do-children-lose-autism-diagnosis.

7. M. J. Maenner et al., "Prevalence of Autism Spectrum Disorder Among Children Aged 8 Years—Autism and Developmental Disabilities Monitoring Network, 11 Sites, United States, 2014," *MMWR Surveillance Summaries* 69, no. SS-4 (March 2020): 1–12. https://doi.org/10.15585/mmwr.ss6706a1.

8. N. M. McDonald et al., "Developmental Trajectories of Infants with Mulitiplex Family Risk for Autism: A Baby Siblings Research Consortium Study," *JAMA Neurology* 77, no. 1 (January 2020): 73–81. https://doi.org/10.1001/jamaneurol.2019.3341.

## Chapter 2

1.  S. Deweerdt, "Regression Marks One in Five Autism Cases, Large Study Finds," Spectrum News, last modified August 17, 2016, https://www.spectrumnews .org/news/regression-marks-one-five-autism-cases-large-study-finds/.

## Chapter 3

1.  "Study Confirms: Autism Wandering Common and Scary," Autism Speaks, last modified August 20, 2018, https://www.autismspeaks.org/news/study -confirms-autism-wandering-common-scary.

## Chapter 9

1.  M. L. Barbera and R. M. Kubina Jr., "Using Transfer Procedures to Teach Tacts to a Child with Autism," *The Analysis of Verbal Behavior* 21, no. 1 (December 2005): 155–161. https://doi.org/10.1007/BF03393017.

## Chapter 10

1.  K. A. Schreck, K. Williams, and A. F. Smith, "A Comparison of Eating Behaviors Between Children With and Without Autism," *Journal of Autism and Developmental Disorders* 34, no. 4 (August 2004): 433–8. https://doi .org/10.1023/b:jadd.0000037419.78531.86.

2.  S. D. Mayes and H. Zickgraf, "Atypical Eating Behaviors in Children and Adolescents with Autism, ADHD, Other Disorders, and Typical Development," *Research in Autism Spectrum Disorders* 64, (2019): 76–83. https://doi.org/10.1016/j.rasd.2019.04.002

# BIBLIOGRAPHY

American Psychiatric Association, *Diagnostic and Statistical Manual of Mental Disorders, 5th Edition: DSM-5.* Washington, D.C.: American Psychiatric Publishing, 2013.

Barbera, Mary. *The Verbal Behavior Approach: How to Teach Children with Autism and Related Disorders.* London: Jessica Kingsley, 2007.

Hodges, Steve J., M.D. *It's No Accident: Breakthrough Solutions to Your Child's Wetting, Constipation, UTIs, and Other Potty Problems.* Guilford, CT: Lyons Press, 2012.

Maurice, Catherine. *Let Me Hear Your Voice: A Family's Triumph Over Autism.* New York: Knopf, 1993.

Skinner, B. F. *Verbal Behavior.* New York: Appleton-Century-Crofts, 1957.

Sundberg, Mark L. *VB-MAPP: Verbal Behavior Milestones Assessment and Placement Program.* Concord, CA: AVB Press, 2008.

Williams, Keith E., and Laura J. Seiverling. *Broccoli Boot Camp: Basic Training for Parents of Selective Eaters.* Bethesda, MD: Woodbine House, 2018.

Williams, Keith E., and Richard M. Fox. *Treating Eating Problems of Children with Autism Spectrum Disorders and Developmental Disabilities.* Austin: Pro-Ed, 2007.

Wirth, Kristen. *How to Get Your Child to Go to Sleep and Stay Asleep,* Victoria, Canada: FriesenPress, 2014.

# INDEX

Note: Page numbers in **bold** reference glossary entries.

## A

ABA. *See* Applied Behavior Analysis (ABA)

ABC (antecedent, behavior, and consequence) data assessment, 79–82, 205, 221

Abstract language concepts, 32, 143–144, 147, 195, 221

ADHD (attention deficit hyperactivity disorder), 2–3, 4–5, 19–20, 185–186, **225**

Advocating for your child, 17, 32, 105, 213–219, 221, 222

Alarms and locks, 37–38

Analysis of Verbal Behavior (Skinner), 6, 8, **229**. *See also Verbal Behavior* (Skinner)

Answering questions (intraverbals), 53, 113–114, 133, 148, **226**

Antecedents, 80–81, 82, 227

Anti-scald device, 40

Anti-tipping cables, 39

Applied Behavior Analysis (ABA)
  advocating for your child when using, 105, 217, 221, 222
  author's personal experience with, 11–12
  defined, **225**
  as early intervention service, 13, 30, 59–60
  as foundation for TAA approach, 6, 8, 12–13. *See also* Turn Autism Around (TAA) approach
  good fit determination and, 96–97
  insurance coverage for, 85, 215–216
  progress and recovery when using, 10, 11, 60, 156, 214–215
  screening tools and, 50, 146

ASD. *See* Autism spectrum disorder

Asperger's syndrome (AS), 22

Assessments, 45–58
  about, 33–34, 45–47, 58, 220; developmental milestone comparison, 47, 50–51, 220; medical information and, 48; for planning purposes, 60–61; screening tools, 9–10, 27, 34, 50, 134, 146, **229**; TAA form, 49–56; video recordings for, 56, 103–104
  of desensitization training, 202
  of eating issues, 48, 152–153, 165
  of imitation skills, 54
  of language skills, 51–54, 56–58, 114–116, 133–134, 138, 146
  of matching skills, 54–55, **227**
  of self-care, 48–51
  of sleeping issues, 48, 170–172
  of social and play skills, 55, 100–101, 102, 103–104
  of tantrums and problem behaviors, 47, 55–56, 79–82, 205, 221, **229**
  of toileting skills, 48, 50, 184–187

Attention deficit hyperactivity disorder (ADHD), 2–3, 4–5, 19–20, 185–186, **225**

Augmentative devices, for communicating, 122

Autism spectrum disorder (ASD)
  author's personal experience, 10–14, 17–18
  "autism" label, 11, 15
  defined, **225**
  as developmental disorder, 2
  diagnosis, 4, 22
  early intervention, importance of, 4–5, 6–10, 13–14, 17–18, 30–32, 59–60. *See also* Turn Autism Around (TAA) approach
  early intervention programs (traditional), 30–32, 59–60, 63–64, 105, 222
  early signs of, 1–2, 12–13. *See also* Signs and symptoms, of autism
  medical issues concurrent with, 16
  normal development and, 19–21

prevalence of, 2–3, 3f
safety issues. *See* Safety issues
sibling and twin studies, 15–16
signs and symptoms of, 19–34. *See also* Signs and symptoms, of autism
wait-and-see approach to, 31
Aversive events. *See* Desensitization training

# B

Babbling, 24, 27, 113, 137
Baseline language sample, 56–58, 114–115
Bathroom behaviors. *See* Toileting skills and interventions
Bathroom safety, 38, 40, 41
Bath time desensitization, 87, 209–210
BCBAs and BCBA-Ds (board certified behavior analysts), 139–140, 151, 214–215, 217–218, **225**
Bedrooms, as place for sleep, 174. *See also* Sleep issues and interventions
"Bedtime" photo album, 177–178
Behavior
    behavioral issues. *See* Tantrums and problem behaviors
    functions of, 77–79
    operant, 113–114, **227**. *See also* Echoics; Intraverbal language; Manding; Tacting
*Behaviors*, of ABC data assessment, 80–81
Body parts, language skills for, 124
Bolting tendencies, 35–36, 40–41, 42–44, 74
Bottle weaning, 159–161, 173–174
Bowel movements
    developmental milestone comparison, 184, 186–187
    interventions for training and wiping, 192, 194–196
    readiness for, 185
Breastfeeding, 158
Bribery vs. reinforcement, 68, 69
Bright lights, 28, 200
*Broccoli Boot Camp* (Williams & Seiverling), 151
Bus safety, 41

# C

Cabinets and drawers, 38

Calendar system documentation, 83–85, 180–182, 187, 205
Carbone, Vincent, 88
Carrier phrases, 139–141
Centers for Disease Control and Prevention (CDC), 33
Chewing issues, 156–157
Colors, 32, 104, 124, 132, 143–144. *See also* Intraverbal language; Pre-academic skills
Community safety issues, 42–44
Conditional discrimination skills, 144, 148
*Consequences*, of ABC data assessment, 81–82
Conversational skills and interventions, 129–148
    about, 129–132; assessment, 133–134, 138, 146; conversation, defined, 132–133; interventions, 138–145, 146–148; materials for, 137; planning, 134–136, 138, 146; progress evaluation, 146
    echoic control development, 137, 142, **226**
    echoics and, 52–53, 113–114, 135, 136–137, **226**
    error fixing and, 138–144
    errorless teaching of, 147–148, **226**
    expressive language and, 144, **226**
    imitation and, 137, **226**
    length of sentences and phrases, 139–141, 147
    as manding, 133, 135
    nonverbal skills and, 144
    pre-academic skill focus mistake, 132, 136, 143–144, 147
    receptive language and, 144
    scripting and, 25, 28, 53, 103–104, 131, 141–142, 146–147, **225, 228**
    transfer trials, 147–148
Cooking safety, 40
Co-sleeping, 167–168, 175
Crib-to-bed transition, 172–173
Crying it out, 8, 31

# D

Daycare, 40–42, 95, 96–97
Declarative pointing, 106
Delayed echolalia (scripting), 25, 28, 53, 103–104, 131, 141–142, 146–147, **225, 228**

# ACKNOWLEDGMENTS

I wasn't planning to write another book since I spent the last several years growing my online courses and community with participants from over 80 countries. But as the members of my toddler course reported amazing progress (within days or weeks in some cases), I knew I needed to write this book and get my Turn Autism Around™ approach out as quickly as possible.

I am grateful to all the parents who trusted me to help their children (in person or online) while I developed my step-by-step approach. I'm especially thankful for the moms who have given me permission to use their stories to help others. It might sound cliché to say "I learned as much from them as they learned from me," but I truly believe that our paths were meant to cross. I am eternally grateful to all the parents and professionals who supported me from the beginning.

To the early supporters of this book, including my online marketing mentor Jeff Walker, who empowered me to think in millions not in thousands and at a magical Durango mastermind, planted the seed for me to write a second book. Jeff and Launch Club members and fellow authors, Ann Sheybani, Walt Hampton, Irina Lee, and Oonagh Duncan, propelled me forward through the book proposal process using their unique gifts and connections.

I'm thankful to Dr. Temple Grandin for agreeing to write the beautiful Foreword and to Melanie Votaw who helped me write the book and get to the finish line!

For the readers of the book drafts, including Kara Renninger, Kathy Henry, Marie Lynch, Rachel Smith, Kelsey General, and Jenna Pethick: your feedback was exceptional!

To my agent Lucinda Blumenfeld who believed in my book and saw the enormous need to get my approach out to the world.

I'd also like to acknowledge my editor Melody Guy, as well as Reid Tracy, Patty Gift, and the entire Hay House team for making the publishing process as easy as possible.

And finally, I'd like to thank my husband, Charles, and my sons, Lucas and Spencer, for encouraging me to pursue my passion and who have been by my side at every step of the journey.

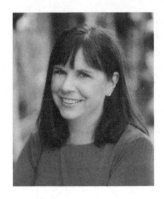

**Mary Lynch Barbera PhD, RN, BCBA-D,** 'fell' into the autism world in the late 1990s when her first-born son, Lucas, started showing signs of autism. Over the past two decades, Mary has transformed from an overwhelmed and confused parent to a doctoral-level Board Certified Behavior Analyst (BCBA-D) and the author of *The Verbal Behavior Approach: How to Teach Children with Autism and Related Disorders.* Mary is an award-winning international speaker, podcaster and online course creator. Her mission is to help parents and professionals turn autism (or signs of autism) around for millions of children around the world.

Websites: MaryBarbera.com and TurnAutismAround.com

# Hay House Titles of Related Interest

*YOU CAN HEAL YOUR LIFE, the movie,*
starring Louise Hay & Friends
(available as an online streaming video)
www.hayhouse.com/louise-movie

*THE SHIFT, the movie,*
starring Dr Wayne W. Dyer
(available as an online streaming video)
www.hayhouse.com/the-shift-movie

\*\*\*

*AWAKENED BY AUTISM: Embracing Autism, Self, and
Hope for a New World,* by Andrea Libutti, M.D.

*ELIMINATING STRESS, FINDING INNER PEACE,* by Brian L. Weiss, M.D.

*EXHAUSTED: How to Revitalize, Restore, and Renew Your Energy,*
by Nick Polizzi and Pedram Shojai, O.M.D.

*THE TAPPING SOLUTION FOR PARENTS, CHILDREN & TEENAGERS:
How to Let Go of Excessive Stress, Anxiety and Worry and Raise Happy,
Healthy, Resilient Families,* by Nick Ortner

*THE WISDOM OF SAM: Observation on Life from an
Uncommon Child,* by Daniel Gottlieb, Ph.D.

All of the above are available at www.hayhouse.co.uk

\*\*\*

# Listen. Learn. Transform.

## Listen to the audio version of this book for FREE!

Unlock endless wisdom, fresh perspectives, and life-changing tools from world-renowned authors and teachers—helping you embrace vibrant health in your body, mind, and spirit. With the *Hay House Unlimited* Audio app, you can learn and grow in a way that fits your lifestyle . . . and your daily schedule.

### With your membership, you can:

- Develop a healthier mind, body, and spirit through natural remedies, healthy foods, and powerful healing practices.

- Explore thousands of audiobooks, meditations, immersive learning programs, podcasts, and more.

- Access exclusive audios you won't find anywhere else.

- Experience completely unlimited listening. No credits. No limits. No kidding.

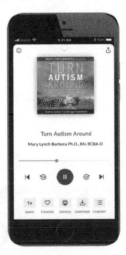

# Try for FREE!

# HAY HOUSE
*Look within*

Join the conversation about latest products,
events, exclusive offers and more.

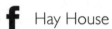 Hay House

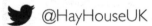 @HayHouseUK

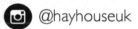 @hayhouseuk

*We'd love to hear from you!*